Critical THINKING TACTICS*
for Nurses
*Tracking, Assessing, and Cultivating Thinking to Improve Competency-Based Strategies

M. Gaie Rubenfeld, RN, MS
Eastern Michigan University
Ypsilanti, MI

Barbara K. Scheffer, RN, EdD
Eastern Michigan University
Ypsilanti, MI

JONES AND BARTLETT PUBLISHERS
Sudbury, Massachusetts
BOSTON   TORONTO   LONDON   SINGAPORE

World Headquarters

Jones and Bartlett Publishers
40 Tall Pine Drive
Sudbury, MA 01776
978-443-5000
info@jbpub.com
www.jbpub.com

Jones and Bartlett Publishers
Canada
6339 Ormindale Way
Mississauga, ON L5V 1J2
Canada

Jones and Bartlett Publishers
International
Barb House, Barb Mews
London W6 7PA
United Kingdom

Jones and Bartlett's books and products are available through most bookstores and online booksellers. To contact Jones and Bartlett Publishers directly, call 800-832-0034, fax 978-443-8000, or visit our website www.jbpub.com.

Substantial discounts on bulk quantities of Jones and Bartlett's publications are available to corporations, professional associations, and other qualified organizations. For details and specific discount information, contact the special sales department at Jones and Bartlett via the above contact information or send an email to specialsales@jbpub.com.

The authors, editor, and publisher have made every effort to provide accurate information. However, they are not responsible for errors, omissions, or for any outcomes related to the use of the contents of this book and take no responsibility for the use of the products and procedures described. Treatments and side effects described in this book may not be applicable to all people; likewise, some people may require a dose or experience a side effect that is not described herein. Drugs and medical devices are discussed that may have limited availability controlled by the Food and Drug Administration (FDA) for use only in a research study or clinical trial. Research, clinical practice, and government regulations often change the accepted standard in this field. When consideration is being given to use of any drug in the clinical setting, the health care provider or reader is responsible for determining FDA status of the drug, reading the package insert, and reviewing prescribing information for the most up-to-date recommendations on dose, precautions, and contraindications, and determining the appropriate usage for the product. This is especially important in the case of drugs that are new or seldom used.

Library of Congress Cataloging-in-Publication Data

Rubenfeld, M. Gaie.
   Critical thinking TACTICS for nurses : Tracking, Assessing, and Cultivating Thinking to Improve Competency-based Strategies / M. Gaie Rubenfeld and Barbara K. Scheffer.
      p. ; cm.
   Includes bibliographical references.
   ISBN 0-7637-4702-5 (alk. paper)
   1. Nursing. 2. Critical thinking.
   [DNLM: 1. Nursing Process. 2. Clinical Competence. 3. Decision Making. 4. Problem Solving. 5. Thinking.
WY 100 R895c 2005] I. Scheffer, Barbara K. II. Title.
   RT42.R78 2005
   610.73—dc22
   6048   2004027911

Production Credits

Acquisitions Editor: Kevin Sullivan
Production Director: Amy Rose
Associate Editor: Amy Sibley
Production Assistant: Alison Meier
Marketing Manager: Emily Ekle

Manufacturing and Inventory Coordinator: Amy Bacus
Composition: Auburn Associates, Inc.
Cover Design: Tim Dziewit
Printing and Binding: Malloy, Inc.
Cover Printing: Malloy, Inc.

Printed in the United States of America
11 10 09 08 07   10 9 8 7 6 5 4 3

This book is dedicated to all nurses—past, present, and future—whose critical thinking often goes unacknowledged for its contribution to keeping us safe and healthy.

Table of Contents

Contributors

Jane Duerr, MSN, APRN, BC, Contributor of clinical scenarios and diligent reviewer.

Mark Steele, Artist, Contributor of cartoon art. www.MarkSteeleArt.com.

Foreword

By Ada Sue Hinshaw, PhD, RN, FAAN, Dean & Professor,
School of Nursing, University of Michigan, Ann Arbor, MI

Explicating and defining the characteristics or habits of the mind and the skills or processes of critical thinking as used in nursing make a unique and valuable contribution to the profession and the discipline. Critical thinking has been a popular buzz phrase in nursing practice and education for a number of years. It has been a central theme for many staff nurse development workshops and for many nursing curricula, especially at the undergraduate level. Yet understanding and explaining the process was very complex and not easily accomplished. The authors started with this basic concern and through their conceptualization and research identified the crucial components delineating the habits or characteristics and skills or processes required of the individual involved in critical thinking.

This text, *Critical Thinking TACTICS for Nurses*, makes a strong contribution to the profession, especially in the practice arenas. The explanations and relationships drawn with critical thinking are laid out in a user-friendly manner that draws on many examples. Through the TACTICS strategy, the professional is led through the critical thinking habits and processes from the perspective of nursing practice. The relationship of critical thinking to evidence-based practice is suggested to be equal, i.e., a professional cannot practice integrating clinical evidence, the latest research, and a career of experience without being involved in critical thinking and all the processes and skills outlined in this text. Understanding these processes and skills empowers the professional nurse for tailoring interventions with clients and ultimately enhances the predictability of the positive outcomes sought for clients and families. Empowering nurses, in terms of their clinical autonomy and control over their practice, has been shown in magnet hospital studies and others to build a stronger, more positive work environment that, in turn, results in better client outcomes through a higher quality of care (McClure & Hinshaw, 2002; IOM, 2004).

Critical thinking occurs within a context. To illustrate how critical thinking relates to several major contextual situations, its relationship and use in patient-centered care, interdisciplinary team care, evidence-based practice, informatics, and quality improvement are outlined. These situations are the five healthcare competencies recommended by the hallmark Institute of Medicine report on *Crossing the Quality Chasm: A New Health System for the 21st Century.* Understanding critical thinking as basic to the attainment of these futuristic competencies is crucial for all health professions, not just nursing.

Critical thinking habits and skills are basic to the conduct of high quality nursing research. Without contextual perspective, creativity, inquisitiveness, intuition, open-mindedness, perseverance, and reflection, few exciting, unique questions would be raised in research. The development of a strong science foundation for nursing practice depends on habits such as contextual perspective, inquisitiveness, and creativity, while the processes and skills such as discriminating, analyzing, and logical reasoning are crucial for scientific inquiry. Transforming knowledge is the skill or process through which research findings are built into practice policies and procedures. Careful attention to critical thinking as part of the undergraduate and graduate nursing curricula prepares nurses for participating in or conducting nursing research, depending on their own career choices.

In both professional practice and in nursing research, the clinical issues confronted and the clinical questions to be investigated are complex and diverse in nature. They require the knowledge and expertise of more than one discipline. Multiple federal reports have recommended interdisciplinary education for the health professions. Critical thinking is basic to all health professions, but a valuable contribution of this text is its explanation of how such thinking is not additive but is greatly expanded when professionals function in interdisciplinary teams either as health providers or investigators.

Rubenfeld and Scheffer are to be commended for explicating what has been a central but conceptually fuzzy entity, i.e., critical thinking. Their research enlightens the nature of both the characteristics or habits and skills or processes involved in such reasoning. Their experience and expertise provide context and practicality. Their contribution to understanding critical thinking as part of or basic to professional practice, research, and education is impressive.

Preface

This book is for clinicians in various practice areas and educators in clinical and academic settings who want to hone their critical thinking abilities and help others do the same. Although written from a nursing perspective, our ideas are applicable in any healthcare discipline.

Healthcare delivery is in dire need of critical thinkers. Although many books and articles note this need, few provide concrete suggestions on how to improve thinking. Most critical thinking (CT) resources are intended for academic audiences. Our aim is to bring critical thinking into the real world of healthcare delivery and education, offering practical suggestions for CT-promoting activities. Note that throughout this book we use the terms "critical thinking" and "thinking" interchangeably. We acknowledge that these terms are not synonymous in other contexts; however, within healthcare, we believe all thinking is critical.

Because CT must be implemented within the context of specific problems or issues, this text addresses the CT needed to achieve five healthcare competencies outlined by the Institute of Medicine (IOM) in its *Quality Chasm* series. These competencies—*patient-centered care, work in interdisciplinary teams, evidence-based practice, using informatics,* and *quality improvement*—will, in the IOM's vision, improve healthcare delivery in the United States. These and very similar competencies have been the foci of healthcare improvement plans in many other countries as well, and the international literature supporting movement in this direction is growing daily. Indeed, we have much to learn from clinicians, researchers, and educators in countries such as Canada, the United Kingdom, Australia, and The Netherlands, especially in the area of evidence-based practice. Informatics has made our world accessible as it never has been before. Not only do we need to work in interdisciplinary teams in our own institutions; teamwork now crosses borders as all nations strive to improve health for their citizens.

Our conceptualization of CT comes from years of practice and research in this area, most notably our Delphi study, which sought to find a consensus description for CT in nursing. Through that research, an expert panel of 55 nurses from 9 countries and 23 US states described 17 dimensions of CT in nursing—10 habits of the mind (affective dimensions) and 7 cognitive skills. The habits of the mind are *confidence, contextual perspective, creativity, flexibility, inquisitiveness, intellectual integrity, intuition, open-mindedness, perseverance,* and *reflection.* The cognitive skills are *analyzing, applying standards, discriminating, information seeking, logical reasoning, predicting,* and *transforming knowledge.* Using these 17 dimensions, CT can be broken down into manageable units, allowing you to see the thinking within the IOM competency contexts.

Keeping a focus on concrete, active learning strategies to promote CT, we employ several practice activities (which we call "TACTICS") in Chapters 1 through 10. These activities help readers reflect on their personal and professional thinking styles while practicing CT-enhancing strategies. Some TACTICS are for educators to use in academic or practice settings; others are directed toward clinicians. Some TACTICS are interchangeable for either educators or clinicians. Chapters 11 and 12 focus on some practical aspects of employing thinking strategies—how to deal with complex change and how to assess CT.

Obviously, this book's title reflects our desire to furnish healthcare providers with practical strategies. TACTICS (Tracking, Assessing, and Cultivating Thinking to Improve Competency-Based Strategies) refers to several activities important to promoting CT. *Tracking* refers to following thinking paths, making them visible and therefore open for study and enhancement. *Assessing* refers to judging the quality of thinking. *Cultivating* refers to a growth-enhancing process; CT is a process, not an end-point. *Thinking,* as mentioned above, is defined as CT with 17 dimensions. *Improve* is just what it says: we want to promote improved CT. *Competency-based strategies* comes from the IOM competencies that serve as the context for our CT discussions. Competency-based refers to performance of CT in the real world rather than an academic checklist. *Strategies* are those means by which CT is practiced and strengthened so that healthcare quality may be enhanced.

In order to provide practical advice to busy clinicians and educators, we have written in short segments and set off specific ideas in prominent boxes, tables, and figures. Although our focus is clearly on thinking, we also need to provide contextual information on a variety of issues. Of necessity, our descriptions of subjects such as informatics, evidence-based practice, and quality improvement are brief and not meant to be primary references on those subjects. And because we appreciate the value of humor in the thinking process, we have enlisted the aid of a superb artist, Mark Steele, to render cartoons to keep you visually stimulated so your thinking stays at its peak and piqued.

We begin this book with a chapter on Frequently Asked Questions, in keeping with our belief that most CT journeys start best with questions. Over the years, as we've conducted numerous workshops and classes on CT, we have been asked many such questions. Chapters 2, 3, 4, and 5 explain the basics of CT in a *what, who, why, how, when,* and *where* format. Chapter 2, "What Is Critical Thinking?", provides the framework of the 17 dimensions, how they were developed, and their distinctive role as one of the few conceptualizations of CT described by nurses and linked to healthcare. Chapter 3, "Who Are the Critical Thinkers?", discusses the importance of individual, cultural, and environmental factors that define us as thinkers. This chapter is specifically intended to address clinicians and educators because it provides various strategies for CT self-reflection. In Chapter 4, "Why Is Critical Thinking So Important?", we explain why CT benefits the many stakeholders in healthcare, especially in terms of safety, effectiveness, and efficiency, and we describe the forces driving the need to focus on CT now. Chapter 5, "The How, When, and Where of Critical Thinking for Clinicians and Educators," introduces the five IOM healthcare competencies as the context for CT. This chapter suggests specific strategies for educators to promote CT in their teaching and strategies for clinicians to actively practice CT.

Chapters 6 through 10 focus on each of the five IOM competencies. Chapter 6, "Critical Thinking and Patient-Centered Care," describes the shift from the old style of provider-centered care and explores how patients and their significant others can use CT in their interactions with providers. Chapter 7, "Critical Thinking and Interdisciplinary Teams," describes the differences between individual and team CT and how both are vital to quality healthcare. Chapter 8, "Critical Thinking and Evidence-Based Practice," explains CT's important role in the shift from basing practice on traditions and authority to one based on the best evidence. Chapter 9, "Critical Thinking and Informatics," explores the burgeoning field of information technology and how CT is essential to health informatics. We especially acknowledge how challenging the rapidly changing field of informatics can be for nurses of our generation in their 40s and 50s. Chapter 10, "Critical Thinking and Quality Improvement," describes the risk-laden state of affairs in healthcare, traces the history of the quality improvement approach, and justifies the need for healthcare reform—reform that we believe should include enhanced CT.

Chapter 11, "Thinking Realities of Yesterday, Today, and Tomorrow," acknowledges the complex changes occurring in healthcare today. We describe the dynamic nature of CT and how it fits perfectly with complex adaptive systems and their constant state of flux. Our final chapter, Chapter 12, explores a popular, but frustrating, topic in nursing—"Assessing Critical Thinking." Clinicians and health educators are being asked to quantify improvements in CT, yet most assessment plans and instruments have been borrowed from other disciplines and have questionable validity in healthcare arenas. Or, they have been created without a clear description of CT or how it works. In this chapter we suggest appropriate assessment methods, including one based on our recent research involving the 17 CT dimensions. This method has proven reliable and efficient, without compromising assessment of all the complexities of CT.

Two appendices supplement the text. The "Critical Thinking Inventory" includes prompts that help people think about their thinking, an essential prerequisite for CT. We have used these prompts successfully for years in our classes and workshops. The second appendix is an "Index of TACTICS" used in this book, so that readers can find them quickly and use them when they will be most beneficial.

We firmly believe that our complex healthcare system has no choice but to change to meet the needs of society today. As clinicians and educators, you must use CT to help bring about those changes and lead the way for the next generation of critical thinkers. These changes must occur if we are to provide higher-quality care in the future.

Because we are primarily educators these days, we enlisted the aid of our nurse practitioner colleague, Jane Duerr, to ensure that we have well-represented clinician perspectives in this book. We hope that her stories from the "swampy lowlands" (to borrow a phrase from Schon) have counterbalanced our ivory tower views. We also hope that you find this book practical and stimulating to your own critical thinking.

Enjoy your thinking journey as you read and reflect. We look to you to continue making CT a natural process within healthcare, today and tomorrow.

Acknowledgments

This book would not have come to life without the assistance of many people. We would like to thank our nursing colleagues who gave us positive feedback on our previous writing projects; without your confidence in our abilities we might not have gone down this path again. Thanks to Dr. George Allen, whose writing expertise we envy; you taught us much about research on critical thinking assessment methods. To Drs. Margaret Lunney and Marsha Fonteyn, who have for years advocated for the importance of critical thinking and supported our work, you remain an inspiration to us. To Dr. Ada Sue Hinshaw, who gave us her valuable time and expertise by writing the foreword for this book, we bow in admiration and thanks.

To our colleagues in practice, we tip our hats in thanks. In particular, we are grateful to Marcia Hegstad, whose daily practice is the epitome of the power of nurses to effect positive change, and Judy Myers, for whom evidence-based practice is as matter of fact as breathing. Thank you both for sharing your experiences with us so that your stories inspire our readers.

We would like to thank our students at Eastern Michigan University who are good-natured about our frequent critical thinking discussions and our creative (sometimes failed) attempts to teach thinking in innovative ways. We especially want to thank David Caraballo for your reflection papers and Jose Valderrama for sharing your Hispanic cultural norms. We would also like to acknowledge the RN-to-BSN students in Monroe, Michigan, who shared numerous insights into their critical thinking while this book was being written.

To Mark Steele, our cartoonist, who constantly amazes us with his ability to capture our ideas in humorous sketches, we say thanks so much for sharing your talents.

To Jane Duerr, our colleague and friend who humbles us with her vast knowledge of nursing practice, we cannot find adequate words to express our gratitude. Your endless hours of editing and help with developing case studies were unbelievably generous, but most of all, we are grateful to you for cheering us on when it looked like we'd never finish this project.

Last, but not least, we'd like to thank our families who tolerate endless hours of viewing only the backs of our heads against the computer screen, who understand our absence from significant events, and who survived our mood swings. We love you and are so grateful that you do the household chores, feed us, run errands, and provide emotional support continually. Jesse, thanks for the pep talks and your artistic inspiration. Tyler, thanks for the hours of computer searching for misplaced references and for your value of writing. Rich, your editing continues to be the expert final hurdle that allows us to think this is good enough to give to the publisher. Nothing would get finished without your help and support. Dan and Anna, Amanda and Ryan, thanks for always asking how things are going with "the book" and offering words of encouragement. Kenn, thanks for helping to find the flow when it was wandering. Thank you Andrew and Allison, whose presence just puts smiles on our faces.

CHAPTER 1

Frequently Asked Questions about Critical Thinking in Nursing

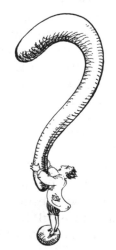

Have you ever asked a question or wondered about critical thinking (CT) in nursing? If so, was your question answered? Most likely, the answer to this question is no or partly. If you are a clinician or an educator, you are aware of the growing number of professional expectations related to CT. It is impossible these days to read accreditation materials or to pick up a nursing textbook without finding some reference to CT as an essential component of healthcare.

We'd like our readers to begin their critical thinking journey with questions for two reasons. First, because that's how we began our travels through the critical thinking maze. Many years ago we asked how we could help nursing students become better thinkers and our exciting exploration of reading, researching, talking, and writing about critical thinking took off. We want to share our discoveries so that you can build on what we have learned. Second,

1

we'd like you to think about your questions, and the questions that they lead to, because they are the essence of great thinking.

The great educational philosopher, Paulo Freire (1998) wrote: "To stimulate questions and critical reflection about the questions, asking what is meant by this or that question, is fundamental to curiosity. Otherwise, all we have is the passivity of students in the face of the discursive explanations of the teacher and answers to questions that have not been asked." (p. 80)

Although we cannot hear your questions, we'd like you to imagine a dialogue with us. Think about your questions and jot down your reflections on them in the margins as you read along. Even though we have been immersed in the teaching of CT in nursing for two decades we probably haven't heard all the possible questions about it. Questions can come from anybody. In the healthcare system alone, nurses, physicians, dieticians, physical therapists, occupational therapists, nursing assistants, technicians, educators, students, legislators, boards of nursing, colleagues from other disciplines, chief nurse executives, patients, and their significant others all ask questions that are relevant and challenging. Because their questions tend to fall into basic categories we have arranged them that way for easy access. And, to make sure our set of questions is as complete as possible, we conducted surveys of practicing nurses and nurse educators, asking them, What is your most burning question about critical thinking in nursing?

Table 1.1 presents the questions organized by category. Following each question is a chapter notation where you can find a relevant discussion, and possibly an answer to the question. If you have questions that are not answered in this text, please feel free to ask us and we will be happy to respond. E-mail your questions to gaie.rubenfeld@emich.edu or bscheffer@emich.edu.

Reference

Freire, P. (1998) *Pedagogy of freedom: Ethics, democracy, and civic courage* (P. Clarke, trans). Lanham, MD: Rowman & Littlefield Publishers, Inc.

Table 1.1   Frequently Asked Questions about Critical Thinking in Nursing

Question category	Questions	Chapter with a response or discussion
Defining and Describing CT	What is CT?	2
	What is CT in nursing? Is it different than in other disciplines?	2
	What's the best definition of CT?	2
	What does CT look like in action?	All
	How do you explain what CT is to a new student or nurse?	2
	What words do you use regularly to represent thinking?	2, App. A
	Why are there so many definitions?	2
	Does it make any difference which definition you pick?	2, 12
	How do you decide what parts of your thinking are the strongest? The weakest?	2, App. A
	Is the CT of women different than the CT of men?	3
	What do "why" questions have to do with CT?	3, 4
	What's the difference between individual CT and team CT?	7
	What's the difference between multidisciplinary team thinking and interdisciplinary team thinking?	7
	What parts of CT are needed for evidence-based practice?	7
	What parts of CT are important for quality improvement?	8
	What kind of thinking is needed for today's healthcare system?	10
	What's so different about individual thinking and systems thinking?	11
		11

(continues)

Table 1.1 Frequently Asked Questions about Critical Thinking in Nursing (continued)

Question category	Questions	Chapter with a response or discussion
Defining and Describing CT (continued)	Is CT just another fad?	All
	Is there research to describe CT?	2
Importance of CT	Why is it important to describe my thinking?	2, 4
	What groups are focusing on CT?	2, 4, 7
	Who in healthcare does CT affect?	All
	Why should administrators and unit managers care about CT?	4
	Why does CT make nursing better?	4
	Why do interdisciplinary teams need CT?	7
	Who thinks interdisciplinary thinking is so important?	7
	Why does the IOM think interdisciplinary thinking is important?	7
	Why is there so much talk about CT with evidence-based practice?	8
	Who is concerned about the thinking needed to improve quality healthcare?	10
	How does thinking about quality affect safe, effective, and efficient care?	10
	How can thinking help us ask better questions?	11
CT in Practice	How does CT affect care planning?	6
	What if I don't have enough time for CT?	11
	What if I'm the only one using CT?	3
	Shouldn't the patient and the family use CT, too?	6
		(continues)

Question	Page
My supervisor told me to think more; what does that mean and how do I do it?	2
What's different about patient's knowledge today that affects CT and the nurse–patient relationship?	6
What helps interdisciplinary teams use team CT?	7
What interferes with CT in interdisciplinary teams?	7
How does evidence-based practice help CT?	8
How can I dispel ideas that evidence-based practice is a cookbook approach that negates CT?	8
How can I figure out which evidence to use?	8
How can I judge clinical guidelines?	8
What do I do if my unit's policies aren't evidence-based and I think we need to change?	8, 11
How can CT help me keep up with the current literature in my practice area?	8, 9
I'm too old for computers; how do I get information to help my CT?	9
Will informatics make nursing harder or easier?	9
How can CT help nurses prevent errors?	10
What does CT have to do with a "culture of safety?"	10
How do you encourage staff to become better critical thinkers?	5, 12
Teaching and Learning CT	
Can CT be taught?	2
How can I describe my thinking to my students?	2, 5
How do I teach CT to people who don't want to think?	2, 5
How can I promote CT in staff and students?	5
How can I be sure I am teaching CT skills?	5, 12
What do you do if your students just don't get it?	5, 12

(continues)

Table 1.1 Frequently Asked Questions about Critical Thinking in Nursing *(continued)*

Question category	Questions	Chapter with a response or discussion
Teaching and Learning CT *(continued)*	What strategies promote CT in the classroom and practice settings?	5, 12
	How can I design assignments that develop CT skills?	5
	How do I incorporate CT skills into the first semester for beginning nursing students?	5
	What activities would increase CT habits of the mind?	5
	Why do I need to teach CT—isn't it just there?	2, 4, 5
	Why is thinking so hard to teach?	4, 5
	Why can't my students and staff just learn to think?	4, 5
	How can I use CT to become a better teacher? A better nurse? A better education coordinator?	4, 5
	When is the best time to start teaching and learning CT skills?	5
	How do I help students see the differences between memorizing and really thinking?	5
	Where is CT best taught, in a classroom or in practice?	5
	How can I promote CT with busy staff nurses?	5, 11
	How can I tell if I'm promoting or blocking thinking?	5, 7, 11
	How can informatics help me teach CT?	9
Measurement of CT	What is the best way to measure CT in students and nurses in the practice setting?	12
	How do I recognize CT when I am reviewing student work?	12
		(continues)

	How do I document the student's progress in CT?	12
	How can informatics help me evaluate CT?	9
	What is the relationship among CT, teaching, and assessment?	5, 12
	How do you measure CT?	12
	What kinds of tests best measure CT?	12
	How can I tell if I'm a good critical thinker?	2, 5, 12
	Can CT be objectively measured?	12
	How can I evaluate CT in staff nurses?	12
	Can I give credit for "partial" CT?	12
Relationship Between CT and Other Things	What is the relationship between CT and NCLEX pass rates?	5
	How can I link clinical experiences with CT?	5
	How does CT fit with JCAHO and the IOM competencies?	4, 5, 10, 11
	What's the difference between critical thinking and clinical judgment?	2
	How do feelings and emotions affect CT?	3
	How is CT affected by self-concept?	3
	How does your perspective on nursing affect CT?	3, 5, 7, 11
	What are the connections between communication skills and CT?	3
	How does the work environment affect CT?	3, 5, 7, 11
	What do IOM competencies have to do with CT?	5, 6–10
	How does CT change the nurse–patient relationship?	6
	How does patient CT affect healthcare team CT?	6, 7, 11
	What is the relationship between evidence-based practice and CT?	8
	What does informatics have to do with CT?	9
	How are CT and quality related?	4, 10
	How does CT fit with complex change?	11

(continues)

Table 1.1 Frequently Asked Questions about Critical Thinking in Nursing *(continued)*

Question category	Questions	Chapter with a response or discussion
Disadvantages of CT	Are there any disadvantages to thinking critically?	11
	How do I avoid being labeled a troublemaker for questioning things?	11
	Does CT make nursing harder?	4
	Are there disadvantages to encouraging patients to be thinking partners?	6
	Why is it so difficult to describe my CT?	2

CHAPTER 2

What Is Critical Thinking?

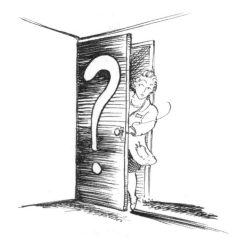

To emphasize the importance of this chapter's question, we will pose some challenges for you. Consider how you would respond to these requests: 1) *describe the thinking you use as a nurse*, 2) *improve your critical thinking*, 3) *tell us what critical thinking is*, 4) *explain how critical thinking is supposed to be practiced in nursing*. We would venture to guess that, even though you consider yourself a good critical thinker, you'd be hard pressed to provide quick, simple responses. And, if you were then asked to describe how you became a nurse who thinks critically, it might be even more challenging. Don't be concerned: first, you're not alone and, second, that's what this book is designed to help you do—help you respond to requests such as those above.

Most people have difficulty describing their thinking processes, even expert clinicians and faculty who teach critical thinking (CT). That's not because they aren't good thinkers; it's just that, until recently, few people asked each other about their thinking and we simply haven't developed a vocabulary to describe such heady things. When asked to describe their thinking, many people pause and say, "I just do!" When pressed to elaborate, you may get a variety of emotional responses. Many people will act frustrated because the request is unusual, they don't have ready answers, and they're too busy to think about it, anyway.

If they're really frustrated, they might respond, Why is it even important to try to describe thinking? Aren't *actions* more important in the big scheme of things? The answer is yes, but actions are only as good as their appropriateness to the problem or condition that prompted the action. In today's healthcare arena those conditions change constantly. What you did yesterday might not work tomorrow or even an hour from now. You must keep abreast of new information and changing patient data and consistently make those things work together. And new information is being discovered and refined daily, if not hourly.

So what is a nurse to do? There's all this existing information, there's a constant flow of new information, and then there's the need to turn it all into a working knowledge so that you can provide safe, effective, efficient nursing actions. You need to bridge the gap between the ever-growing information and the actions it requires. You need a series of steps or a process to convert information into knowledge. Finally, you must translate that knowledge, which is very abstract, into practice actions, which are very concrete. That transition works best if you can recognize those steps or processes; otherwise you are less likely to arrive at predictable and consistently successful actions.

We can't all be like Indiana Jones in the movie *Indiana Jones and the Last Crusade*. He stepped off into the chasm as a leap of faith. After he found himself on firm footing, he threw pebbles back to define the bridge that was camouflaged by its surroundings. Think of critical thinking as that bridge. We will provide some pebbles ahead of time; once you see that critical thinking bridge your mind will more easily transform information into knowledge and that knowledge, albeit abstract, will be the basis of the best workable course of action. *Why* this is so important will be addressed in Chapter 4 but, for now, we need you to accept on faith that it's worth your while to understand *what* we're talking about when we use the term CT.

THE CRITICAL THINKING "BRIDGE"

So CT is the metaphorical bridge between information and action, but what are those pebbles for? They're going to do for you exactly what they did for Indiana Jones: they're going to turn something that is invisible from one perspective into something visible from a new perspective. But first, it might be helpful to look at the three reasons why the bridge (CT) is invisible in the first place. Reason Number 1: **CT is intangible**; you can't study it under a microscope, hold it, smell it, examine it for a pulse. Reason Number 2: **CT is very individual**—no two people think in the same way, nor do they broadcast their thoughts, so it's impossible to learn how to think critically by watching only actions. Reason Number 3: **CT requires effort**. Many of us assume CT will just happen over time as we gain knowledge and experience, so we just wait and don't worry about it. This may have worked in the past but time is a luxury these days. We need to use CT today, not tomorrow.

So how can you start to see this previously invisible CT? Can you do it without pebbles? To some extent, yes, you probably can. For example, think about the opposite of CT. We'll bet you can easily identify people who don't use CT. What do they do? Now think of a nurse you consider to be a great thinker. She's the person you want to work with, especially if you're a novice. If something new comes up, she's the one who can figure out how to deal with it. She's creative, open-minded, logical. Now, with this positive image, the next question is can *you* learn to get to that expert level of thinking? How and how quickly? Can you help other nurses get there, too? The good news is yes, you can. However, this is where the pebbles come in. The pebbles are the three tools that will make the process of becoming a great critical thinking nurse easier.

PEBBLES ON THE METAPHORICAL BRIDGE

First, you need to be clear on just what CT in nursing is—for that you need a definition. Second, you need to know how to describe what "it" looks like, using words to elaborate on the definition. Both of these tasks require a vocabulary. Once you can use specific words to describe your thinking processes, you can more easily discover what you're good at and where you need to improve. With a definition and words you can also help others identify, describe, and improve their critical thinking. Third, you will need to visualize what CT words look like in action, particularly as CT is practiced in nursing. Addressing these three points—a definition, a vocabulary, and translating words to actions—will help us figure out the *what* of CT.

Pebble #1: Defining CT

Let's start by tackling the issue of defining and describing CT in nursing. We can't do justice to that task without some contextual and historical perspective. There are many descriptions of critical thinking in the literature; however, because many of those definitions are borrowed from other disciplines they vary in terms of usefulness to nursing. We'll discuss some of the problems with those definitions in Chapter 12. For now, let's focus on the historical context of CT so that you can appreciate how essential this concept is to ourselves, to our patients, our students, and our society.[1]

In Western history, CT can be traced back to Socrates and his Socratic Method, or answering questions with questions. Actually, Socrates emphasized deep questioning of ideas that were accepted as fact, but which may simply have been beliefs. For example, everyone then believed the earth was flat but this did not make it a fact. Later, Plato and Aristotle expanded on Socrates' ideas to emphasize that things are not always what they seem and that sound reasoning takes into account objections to accepted ideas. During the Renaissance, Francis Bacon focused on empirical information gathering, establishing our modern research standards of systematic study. That empirical, or fact, base was important to overcome the natural biases that our minds use to understand our world and our place in it. René Descartes promoted systematic doubt: all thinking should be questioned and tested. (It may be comforting to those who spend lots of time thinking about thinking that Descartes acknowledged our existence as thinking beings to be the most factual thing to know. Even if we doubt that anything else exists, *we must exist* to do the doubting. Now, think about that!) In the 18th century Immanuel Kant's *Critique of Pure Reason* examined the conundrum of using principles for thinking that cannot be empirically tested. Consider this statement: We are "burdened by questions . . . prescribed by . . . reason itself . . . [which we] are not able to ignore, but which . . . [we are] also not able to answer" (1965, p. 7).

John Dewey, the often cited CT promoter in educational circles, took CT into the 20th century with his pragmatic view of thought as part of human behavior. We'll revisit his ideas in Chapter 5. And Jean Piaget, cautioning about the dangers of egocentric and sociocentric characteristics of human thought, emphasized the need to be open to multiple points of view. In the 1980s, the aviation industry began designing strategies to help pilots progress from novice to expert levels more quickly (Dreyfus & Dreyfus, 1986). That industry was very interested in the CT of human pilots because an aircraft's autopilot could not be programmed to react to all the dynamic events that occur when taking off, flying, and landing an airplane. As advanced as artificial intelligence is, it cannot yet replace the human thinking required in emergency situations. Patricia Benner (1984), a well-known

---

[1]With our apologies to the historians and philosophers in our audience who are already aware of this history, we will give only a quick overview of CT's philosophical roots. For those of you who yearn for more, check out some philosophy books or go to this website that we used for much of the information in this section: http://www. philosophypages.com (Kemerling, 2002). Being Westerners, we will also apologize to other cultures, such as those from Asia, whose CT roots could be traced, for example, to the teaching of Lao Tzu or Confucius.

nursing theorist, collaborated with Dreyfus and Dreyfus in the development of her Novice to Expert Model of nursing care. It is not surprising that the aviation industry and professional nursing are equally concerned about critical thinking—both deal with split second decision making to keep people safe.

Thinking, how the brain works, and how learning takes place became dominant themes in education in Western society in the early 1980s (Hart, 1983). Initially, the focus was on teaching CT in kindergarten through grade 12, with books such as *Developing Minds: A Resource Book for Teaching Thinking* (Costa, 1985). In the early 1990s the movement to improve thinking spread to post secondary education. Assessment of all students' CT skills is now part of college and university accreditation standards in the United States. For example, criterion 4 of *the Higher Learning Commission's "Institutional Accreditation Guidelines"* (2003) cited the importance of "fostering and supporting inquiry, creativity, practice and social responsibility" (pdf p. 6).

Also during the 1990s, critical thinking became a focus in nursing education. The National League for Nursing Accrediting Commission (NLN-AC) has cited CT as an expected program outcome. Programs currently accredited by NLN-AC are expected to include and assess critical thinking in their curricula (2003). The American Association of Colleges of Nursing (AACN) also emphasizes CT as a core competency. Its *Essentials of Baccalaureate Education for Professional Nursing Practice* (1998) provides a brief description of CT, and its accreditation arm—the Commission on Collegiate Nursing Education (CCNE)—requires nursing programs to address all of the components in the *Essentials* document, including CT (2003).

Thinking became a theme in healthcare delivery as well. The Joint Commission on Accreditation of Healthcare Organizations (JCAHO) first developed standards mandating competency assessment and documentation in the healthcare arena in the early 1990s (2000). Competency-focused care requires clinicians and staff development specialists to hone their CT skills. In Case's (1998) "Competence Development: Critical Thinking, Clinical Judgment, and Technical Ability," staff development specialists were given practical strategies for nurturing CT. We will elaborate on the subject of competency and CT in Chapter 5. The American Nurses' Association (ANA) also emphasizes CT in its current *Nursing: Scope and Standards of Practice*. The language of CT is addressed in the association's scope statement and incorporated throughout all of the standards (2003). Nurse leaders have increasingly recognized the importance of thinking skills in nursing but to guide this change transformational leadership, supported by evidence-based management at all levels of administration, is needed (Thomson & Burns, 2004; Miller et al., 2001; Hansten & Washburn, 1999; IOM, 2004; Schoenly, 1998).

Outside of healthcare clinical settings, a seminal work by the American Philosophical Association (APA), under the direction of Facione, defined CT using a Delphi method to survey academicians. Philosophers composed roughly half of his 46-member panel; others were from fields such as education, physics, computer science, and psychology. They arrived at this consensus statement: "We understand critical thinking to be purposeful, self-regulatory judgment which results in interpretation, analysis, evaluation, and inference as well as explanation of the evidential, conceptual, methodological, criteriological, or contextual considerations upon which judgment is based" (1990, p. 2). This definition of CT has been used extensively in nursing but, because no nurses or healthcare providers participated in the APA study, there is some question as to whether it's findings are the best fit for nursing.

Because of the growing need for CT in nursing, some practitioners found it necessary to develop nursing-specific conceptualizations of CT so we could teach it better (e.g., Rubenfeld & Scheffer, 1999). In recent years, nurses have used research to describe CT and its components so that we have stronger evidence of CT in our profession. Of note is Fonteyn's (1998) work to describe thinking strategies for nursing practice. Using a "think aloud" method, Fonteyn and her team studied 14 expert registered nurses from a variety of specialty areas. Twelve predominant thinking strategies were identified. See Box 2.1.

Following a method similar to that used by Facione for the APA, we conducted a comprehensive study to find consensus on a description of critical thinking in nursing in the mid 1990s (Scheffer & Rubenfeld, 2000). In this three-year study, we also employed a Delphi method to gain consensus from a

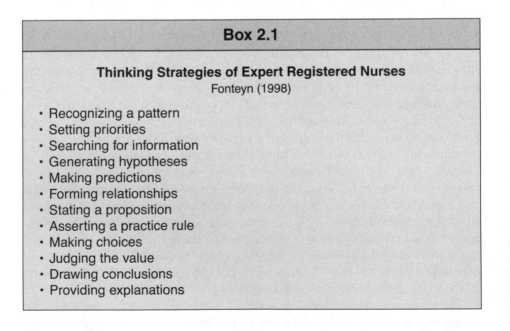

Box 2.1

Thinking Strategies of Expert Registered Nurses
Fonteyn (1998)

- Recognizing a pattern
- Setting priorities
- Searching for information
- Generating hypotheses
- Making predictions
- Forming relationships
- Stating a proposition
- Asserting a practice rule
- Making choices
- Judging the value
- Drawing conclusions
- Providing explanations

geographically disperse group of expert nurses through successive rounds of questions, answers, data analysis, and voting (Goodman, 1987). Our panel of 55 expert nurses was called from practice, education, and research settings, from nine countries and 23 US states, and during five rounds of questions and responses, we identified and defined ten habits of the mind and seven cognitive skills of critical thinking in nursing.

We started our consensus rounds with a broad question: What are the skills and habits of the mind of critical thinking in nursing? Our choice of words was deliberate: we wanted to get at not only the cognitive skills, but the affective component as well. Numerous authors (e.g., Tanner, 1997) have identified the importance of this affective component, which Facione (1990) named "dispositions." After a most helpful discussion with Dr. Pete Facione (a philosopher–scholar) and his wife, Dr. Noreen Facione (a nurse–scholar), we chose the label "habits of the mind" because we wanted to get away from some of the stereotypical views of traits or dispositions as being static. Since habits can be initiated and changed, this term seemed to be more dynamic.

Throughout the rounds of our Delphi process we "analyzed" data and returned reports to participants explaining what we had done with their information and asking a new set of questions based on the revised configuration of the data. By the end of five rounds we were ready for voting on the final statement and definitions of the 10 habits of the mind and seven skills. There was 88.2% consensus on the final statement and similar consensus on the definitions of the dimensions. (For the full report of the research method and consensus voting see Scheffer & Rubenfeld, 2000). The final consensus statement is:

> Critical thinking in nursing is an essential component of professional account-ability and quality nursing care. Critical thinkers in nursing exhibit these habits of the mind: confidence, contextual perspective, creativity, flexibility, inquisitive-ness, intellectual integrity, intuition, open-mindedness, perseverance, and reflec-tion. Critical thinkers in nursing practice the cognitive skills of analyzing, apply-ing standards, discriminating, information-seeking, logical reasoning, predicting and transforming knowledge (p. 357).

See Box 2.2 and the tear-out card on the inside cover of this book for defini-tions of the 10 habits of the mind and seven skills. These dimensions of CT in nursing will be used as a framework for discussing CT throughout this text, so you will want to be able to refer to them frequently.

Comparison of the Nursing Delphi Study to the Philosophical Delphi Study

Box 2.3 compares the results of our study with those of Facione and his group. The definitions of CT skills are from Facione's 1990 Delphi study. The

Box 2.2

Critical Thinking Skills and Habits of the Mind for Nursing
(Scheffer and Rubenfeld, 2000, p. 358: used with permission.)

Critical Thinking SKILLS

Analyzing: separating or breaking a whole into parts to discover their nature, function and relationships

Applying Standards: judging according to established personal, professional or social rules or criteria

Discriminating: recognizing differences and similarities among things or situations and distinguishing carefully as to category or rank

Information Seeking: searching for evidence, facts or knowledge by identifying relevant sources and gathering objective, subjective, historical and current data from those sources

Logical Reasoning: drawing inferences or conclusions that are supported in or justified by evidence

Predicting: envisioning a plan and its consequences

Transforming Knowledge: changing or converting the condition, nature, form or function of concepts among contexts

Critical Thinking Habits of the Mind

Confidence: assurance of one's reasoning abilities

Contextual Perspective: considerate of the whole situation, including relationships, background and environment, relevant to some happening

Creativity: intellectual inventiveness used to generate, discover, or restructure ideas; imagining alternatives

Flexibility: capacity to adapt, accommodate, modify or change thoughts, ideas and behaviors

Inquisitiveness: an eagerness to know by seeking knowledge and understanding through observation and thoughtful questioning in order to explore possibilities and alternatives

Intellectual Integrity: seeking the truth through sincere, honest processes, even if the results are contrary to one's assumptions and beliefs

Intuition: insightful sense of knowing without conscious use of reason

Open-mindedness: a viewpoint characterized by being receptive to divergent views and sensitive to one's biases

(continues)

Box 2.2 *(continued)*

Perseverance: pursuit of a course with determination to overcome obstacles

Reflection: contemplation upon a subject, especially one's assumptions and thinking for the purposes of deeper understanding and self-evaluation

Box 2.3

Comparison of Nursing and APA Components of CT

Nursing Skills
(Scheffer & Rubenfeld, 2000, p. 358)

APA Skills
(Facione, 1990)

Analysis:
"to identify the intended and actual inferential relationships among statements, questions, concepts, descriptions or other forms of representation intended to express beliefs, judgments, experiences, reasons, information, or opinions" (p. 14). Its subskills are identified as "examining ideas, identifying arguments and analyzing arguments" (p. 12)

Analyzing:
"separating or breaking a whole into parts to discover their nature, function and relationships"

Applying Standards:
"judging according to established personal, professional or social rules or criteria"

Evaluation:
"to assess the credibility of statements or other representations which are accounts or descriptions of a person's perception, experience, situation, judgment, belief, or opinion; and to assess the logical strength of the actual or intended inferential relationships among statements, descriptions, questions or other form of representation" (p. 15)

(continues)

Box 2.3 (continued)

Discriminating:
"recognizing differences and similarities among things or situations and distinguishing carefully as to category or rank"

Information Seeking:
"searching for evidence, facts or knowledge by identifying relevant sources and gathering objective, subjective, historical and current data from those sources"

Logical Reasoning:
"drawing inferences or conclusions that are supported in or justified by evidence"

Predicting:
"envisioning a plan and its consequences"

Transforming Knowledge:
"changing or converting the condition, nature, form or function of concepts among contexts"
No comparable skill; see Habit of the Mind, Reflection.

Interpretation:
"to comprehend and express the meaning or significance of a wide variety of experiences, situations, data, events, judgments, conventions, beliefs, rules, procedures or criteria" (p. 13)
(Its sub-skills are *categorization, decoding sentences* and *clarifying meaning.*)

Inference sub-skill:
querying evidence:
"to identify and secure elements needed to draw reasonable conclusions" (p. 16)

Explanation:
"to state the results of one's reasoning; to justify that reasoning in terms of the evidential, conceptual, methodological, criteriological and contextual considerations upon which one's results were based; and to present one's reasoning in the form of cogent arguments" (p. 18)

Inference sub skill:
conjecturing alternatives: "to formulate multiple alternatives for resolving a problem . . . to draw out presuppositions and project the range of possible consequences of decisions, positions, policies, theories, or beliefs"
(p. 17)
No comparable skill

Self-regulation

(continues)

| Box 2.3 *(continued)* |

Nursing Habits of the Mind
(Scheffer & Rubenfeld, 2000, p. 358)

APA Dispositions
(Facione, Sanchez, Facione, & Gainen, 1995)

CT Self-Confidence:
"to trust the soundness of one's own reasoned judgments and to lead others in the rational resolution of problems" (p. 8)

Confidence:
"assurance of one's reasoning abilities"

Contextual Perspective:
"considerate of the whole situation, including relationships, background and environment, relevant to some happening"

Maturity:
"approach[ing] problems, inquiry, and decision making with a sense that some problems are necessarily ill-structured, some situations admit more than one plausible option, and many times judgments must be made based on standards, contexts, and evidence which preclude certainty" (p. 9)

Flexibility:
"capacity to adapt, accommodate, modify or change thoughts, ideas and behaviors"

No comparable disposition

Creativity:
"intellectual inventiveness used to generate, discover, or restructure ideas; imagining alternatives"

Inquisitiveness: "an eagerness to know by seeking knowledge and understanding through observation and thoughtful questioning in order to explore possibilities and alternatives"

Inquisitiveness:
"one's intellectual curiosity and one's desire for learning even when the application of the knowledge is not readily apparent" (p. 6)

Intellectual Integrity:
"seeking the truth through sincere, honest processes, even if the results are contrary to one's assumptions and beliefs"

Truthseeking:
"being eager to seek the best knowledge in a given context, courageous about asking questions, and honest and objective about pursuing inquiry even if the findings do not support one's self-interests or one's preconceived opinions" (p. 8)

(continues)

Box 2.3 *(continued)*	
Intuition: insightful sense of knowing without conscious use of reason	*No comparable disposition*
Open-mindedness: a viewpoint characterized by being receptive to divergent views and sensitive to one's biases	*Open-mindedness:* "being tolerant of divergent views and sensitive to the possibility of one's own bias" (p. 6)
Perseverance: pursuit of a course with determination to overcome obstacles	*Systematicity:* "being organized, orderly, focused and diligent in inquiry" (p. 7)
Reflection: contemplation upon a subject, especially one's assumptions and thinking for the purposes of deeper understanding and self-evaluation	*No comparable disposition but comparable to APA skill: Self-Regulation:* "self-consciously to monitor one's cognitive activities, the elements used in those activities, and the results educed, particularly by applying skills in analysis and evaluation to one's own inferential judgments with a view toward questioning, confirming, validating, or correcting either one's reasoning or one's results" (Facione, 1990, p. 19)
No comparable habit of the mind.	*Analyticity:* "prizing the application of reasoning and the use of evidence to resolve problems, anticipating potential conceptual or practical difficulties, and consistently being alert to the need to intervene" (p. 7)

dispositions descriptions are taken from Facione, Sanchez, Facione and Gainen (1995). In Facione's original work, he found 19 dispositions that fit into two types—approaches to life and living in general, and approaches to specific issues, questions, or problems. Those 19 dispositions were later consolidated to form seven dispositions in a factor analysis by Facione, Facione, and Sanchez (1994) as they began to develop a CT dispositions test.

While the comparisons are not direct, there are striking similarities between the two study results. However, a significant difference is also apparent. Two habits of the mind and one skill were not identified by the APA group—*creativity*, *intuition*, and *transforming knowledge*. Are these dimensions unique to nursing? Or are they unique to applied sciences or to health professions? We believe that our comparison shows that there are quite likely some discipline-specific dimensions of CT and some that are possibly universal.

Pebble #2: CT Language/Words

If these 17 dimensions represent CT in nursing, let's see how your thinking fits with them. Think about your thinking. Ask yourself, for example, how strong is your critical thinking *confidence* or how do you use *analyzing* in your clinical practice.

TACTICS 2.1: CT Self-Checklist

Look at Box 2.4 and mark where you think you fall on each of those thinking continua.

This TACTIC can be used by both clinicians and educators.

Box 2.4
Critical Thinking Self-Checklist

1. How confident am I in my reasoning ability?
   Not very confident   Very confident
2. Do I tend to look at situations with their context in mind or do I tend to see things as separate compartments?
   Compartmentalized thinking   Contextual thinking
3. How creative am I in my thinking?
   Not very creative   Very creative
4. How flexible is my thinking?
   Rigid   Very flexible
5. How inquisitive am I?
   Not naturally curious   Innately inquisitive
6. How much intellectual integrity do I have?
   Go with my assumptions   Seek the truth no matter what
7. How intuitive am I?
   Not very intuitive   Always go with my gut

(continues)

Box 2.4 *(continued)*

---

8. How open-minded am I?
   Quite biased   Open to all possibilities

9. How much perseverance do I have in my thinking?
   Once I have problems I'll stop   Keep at it no matter what gets in
                                       the way

10. How reflective am I? Do I think about my thinking?
    Not very reflective   Always striving for deeper under-
                                       standing of self

11. How good am I at analyzing situations?
    I don't break things down much   I always pick things apart to
                                       understand them

12. How much do I pay attention to standards with my thinking?
    Not used much for judgments   Always use criteria for judgments

13. How finely do I discriminate among things?
    Don't recognize small   Always recognize small things
    differences/similarities

14. How good am I at seeking out information?
    I think about what's right there   I dig for all possible evidence

15. How strong is my logical reasoning?
    I can't always justify my   I can always trace my conclu-
    conclusions   sions to evidence

16. How good are my abilities to predict consequences in situations?
    Don't see much farther than   I always think what would happen
    my nose   if

17. How well do I transform knowledge from one situation to the next?
    Prefer textbook situations   Can adapt concepts to meet
                                       situation

Discussion

Are you beginning to see where your strengths and weaknesses lie? Let's take this further. At the beginning of this chapter we asked how you would describe the thinking you use. Now how would you describe your thinking? Is it different now that you have the words to use? Is it easier to describe your thinking now that you know the words? Have you ever had to do this? In fact, most of us haven't been asked to describe our thinking—at least not until recently. These days clinicians are being asked to show how they think because CT is recognized as being tied to quality of care. We need a new language of thinking—and a mutual understanding of what the words in that language mean.

Do you remember the first time you used a computer, ran into problems, and asked for help? If your helper was like most computer-literates, she probably used words like *booting, DOS, windows,* and *right click.* Did you sit there with your mouth hanging open feeling foolish? Were you at a loss to say anything because you didn't know the language? Eventually, you probably learned enough computer lingo to function in today's technological world. Well, learning how to describe CT is a similar process. Without the words it's impossible to even ask useful questions.

When we first started to teach CT, when we asked students to describe how they were thinking, they would tell us *what* they were thinking about. After trying several tactics to get our point across, we finally realized the communication problem was very basic. Very few of our students had a vocabulary to use; they were not accustomed to describing something so abstract. As we used words to describe CT in nursing more and more in class, eventually it became clear that a list of descriptors would help students describe their thinking. Look at Box 2.5 and see how many of those words and phrases you use and when and where you've heard or seen others using them.

Box 2.5

Words to Describe Critical Thinking
Descriptors for CT Habits of the Mind

Confidence
My thinking was on track, decisive; I reconsidered and still thought I made the best decision; I knew my conclusion was well-founded; My thinking was clear, unambiguous, trustworthy; I was secure in my thinking

Contextual Perspective
I could see the whole picture; I considered [reflected on, reconsidered] other possibilities; I took other things [surrounding issues] under consideration; I redefined the situation in view of; Considering the circumstances, I . . . ; I broadened my view/perspective/mind

Creativity
I let my imagination go; I was inspired to think of; I stretched my mind; I took my thinking outside the box; I envisioned/dreamed up/invented; I tried to be visionary; My mind was fertile ground; I used the artistic side of my brain

(continues)

Box 2.5 *(continued)*

Flexibility
I changed directions in my mind; I gave up on that idea and went on to; I moved away from my traditional thinking; I redefined the situation and started again; I questioned what I was thinking and considered another path; I tried to be adaptable in my thinking; I let my thinking go with the flow

Inquisitiveness
I had a strong desire for more knowledge; I itched to know more about; I was eager to know more; I took a lively interest in; I pricked up my ears, stuck my nose in; I burned with curiosity; I was really interested in; My mind was buzzing with questions

Intellectual Integrity
I was not satisfied with my conclusion so I; Although it went against everything I believed; I need to get at the truth; I tried to find the bottom line; I racked my brain; I questioned my biases; I asked myself difficult questions; I dug to the bottom; I reflected on my inferences; I examined why I thought that

Intuition
I felt it in my bones; I couldn't put my finger on why, but I thought; Instinctively I knew; My hunch was that; I had a premonition/inspiration/impression; My natural tendency was to; Subconsciously I knew that; Without thought I figured out; Automatically I thought that; While I couldn't say why, I thought immediately; My sixth sense said I should consider

Open-mindedness
I tried to be receptive to new ideas; I tried not to judge; I listened to reason; I looked at both sides of the issue; I tried to be objective and unprejudiced; I questioned why I thought that; I weighed the pros and cons; I tried to be neutral

Perseverance
I was single-minded in my determination to; I persistently kept at it; I plodded on through my thoughts; I was stubborn and tireless in my pursuit; I kept going, trying this and that; I would not accept that for an answer; I had to overcome so many obstacles

Reflection
I pondered my reactions; I mulled it over in my mind; I ruminated over what I had thought and done; I had to reexamine/rethink/reconsider/review things; I evaluated my thoughts; I wondered what I could have done differently; I concentrated on my thinking process; I talked to myself about; I deliberately meditated on what I was thinking

(continues)

Box 2.5 *(continued)*

Descriptors for CT Skills

Analyzing

I dissected the situation; I broke things down so I could understand them better; I tried to reduce things into manageable units; I detailed a schematic of; I sorted things out; I took the whole situation apart so I could see; I looked for the parts; I made sure each component was addressed; I set it out, one, two, or three; I looked at each piece individually; I studied it bit by bit; I thought of it piecemeal instead of all together; I tried to see the trees instead of just the forest

Applying Standards

I knew I had to; There are certain things you just have to account for; I thought of the bottom line that is always; I know that some things are just right or wrong; As a professional, I knew I had to; I knew it was unethical to; I considered what my license allowed and expected me to do; I thought of/studied the policy for; I compared this situation to what I knew to be the rule; I judged that according to

Discriminating

I grouped things together; I put things in categories; I tried to consider what was the priority; I rank ordered the various; I stood back and tried to see how those things were related; I wondered if this was as important as; I thought of the discrepancies in the story; I could distinguish the pieces; What I was hearing and what I was seeing was consistent [inconsistent]; I wondered what I should do first; When I focused on the finer details, I could see; This was different from [the same as] that

Information Seeking

I made sure I had all the pieces of the picture; I knew I needed to look up/study; I wondered how I could find out; I went back to look more closely at; I asked myself if I knew the whole story; I kept searching for more data; I wanted [needed] to have all the facts [knowledge]; I looked for evidence of

Logical Reasoning

I deduced from the information that; I could trace my conclusion back to the data; My diagnosis was grounded in the evidence; I considered all the information and then inferred; I could justify my conclusion by; I moved down a straight path from initial data to the final conclusion; I had a strong argument for; I made a good case for; There was sound evidence to support; My rationale for the conclusion was; Putting two and two together I inferred; I brought reason to bear in the situation by

(continues)

Box 2.5 *(continued)*
Predicting I could imagine that happening if I did; I anticipated; I was prepared for; I tried to be farsighted in my view; I made provisions for; I envisioned the outcome to be; I had a feeling that would happen; I could foresee; My prognosis was; I figured the probability of; I could tell that down the line; I tried to go beyond the here and now; The immediate plan was this, but the long term needed to be ***Transforming Knowledge*** I knew I'd have to individualize; Although this situation was somewhat different, I knew; I wondered if that would fit in this situation; I thought this would be a textbook case but it wasn't; I took what I knew and asked myself if it would work; I tried to translate that into this; I adapted my knowledge about; I could accommodate; I improved on the basics by adding; I figured if this was true then that would be too; At first I was puzzled; then I saw that there were similarities, too; It was easy to cross over

If you think you're ready, you can go to Appendix A and look at the CT Inventory. It's a more detailed version of the checklist in Box 2.4 and can be used in a variety of situations. (You may find the descriptors in Box 2.5 helpful when answering the questions it poses.) This inventory has been used to help nurses and nursing students describe their thinking and to evaluate growth in CT. Once you take the time to complete that inventory, we think you'll have a better sense of how you think and you would really be able to answer someone who asked, How would you describe your thinking as a nurse?

If, at this point, you are really excited by CT, you can tease your brain by considering the CT Ironies in Box 2.6. If you can spend enjoyable time pondering these more esoteric points, you have the makings of a philosopher!

Box 2.6
CT Ironies to Ponder
• If I teach you what CT is, I'm actually discouraging you from using CT to figure it for yourself. • If I argue that CT is impossible or unnecessary, I'm actually being contradictory since posing such argumentation demonstrates CT. • If CT truly requires a contextual perspective, then I must always adapt to the context to promote CT; does then CT itself change per context?

Pebble #3: Visualizing CT in Action

And now for CT in action. What does it look like? *Can* you see it? Some argue that we cannot see or measure CT because it is only manifested in actions. That is somewhat true, but there are problems with just looking at actions. Some "right" actions are pure luck; you can't count on them happening the next time. Some "right" actions are based on sloppy thinking. And some "right" actions are based on keen CT. Which kind of thinking do you want to count on? Sometimes it's easier to see the consequences of not thinking well than to see the results of well-thought-out actions. Things go wrong when nurses don't use CT. To fully appreciate CT in action, one really needs to combine descriptions of thinking with the actions that thinking produces. The following TACTICS illustrate that combined approach.

TACTICS 2.2: What Do Great Thinkers Look Like?

Clinicians

Think of the people you work with; rank them in terms of their thinking. One or two people probably stand out as great thinkers. What makes you put them in the great-thinker category? It's probably their actions and their communication. Now, list those characteristics and see if you can picture great thinking in action.

Educators

Have your students or staff do the exercise above, writing down their descriptions of a great thinker they know personally, either as a formal paper or as an informal list of characteristics. Then have them share their descriptions and look for commonalities.

Discussion

In our workshops, students who do this exercise report the characteristics of great thinkers as: This person "always explains what he's doing . . . is always asking questions . . . can always stand up for herself when she's questioned . . . teaches every patient and family member he comes in contact with . . . rarely takes things at face value . . . rechecks everything . . . is the one we all go to for help with medication calculations . . . says what's on her mind . . . is the one we like to work with."

TACTICS 2.3: Talking and Thinking—a Patient Scenario

Clinician

Consider this scenario. You are working on a medical unit. Mrs. Franks, 79 years old with a history of alcoholism, was admitted two days ago for heart failure. Two hours before your shift began, she was moved to your unit from the telemetry unit. According to your shift report, she has been alert and oriented, has some minor lower extremity edema, has gone from many to a few crackles in her lungs, had her Foley removed this morning, and has urinated once in the past six hours. Her weight has decreased 4 kg since admission. She is not on a fluid restriction and has been eating and drinking small amounts. She has used her prn oxygen rarely. You walk into the room to find a very agitated Mrs. Franks trying to get out of bed, saying, "I have to get to the store before it closes because I have company coming for dinner." Speaking in a calm voice you ask her to tell you how she feels. Meanwhile you check her pulse and find it at 92 but regular. You remember that she's on a beta-blocker . . .

Now, finish this scenario. What would you think? What would you do and why?

Educators

Use this same case or find one that works with your setting and matches the level of knowledge of your students or staff. Service-based educators should select a unit-specific case. Set up some parameters for responding to this scene; for example, if you are trying to promote better assessment skills among one unit's staff, have the nurses list their answers and place them in a centrally located box for a drawing later. Give a prize for the best answer or post all the answers anonymously and have the staff rate them.

Discussion

So, what would exemplify best thinking in this situation with Mrs. Franks? We'll give you an idea of what an expert nurse would do. Obviously, novices would not necessarily come up with these responses.

We'd expect the nurse to assess: respiratory rate, lung sounds, pulse oximetry, blood pressure, temperature, cognitive function, glucose (if there's any history of hypo or hyper glycemia), hemoglobin level to consider if she's anemic, medications and side effects, additional information about her alcoholism (e.g., how long since drinking last, amount consumed), and her past history of alcoholic behavior, via her chart or family report, if possible. We'd also want the nurse to check patterns to see if her pulse of 92 is normal according to her baseline.

We'd expect each of those things to be assessed in just about that order. We'd expect the nurse to speak softly and confidently to the patient, ask her if she needs the bathroom or is in pain, orient her to her surroundings, help her stay in bed, and make sure she is safe before leaving the patient alone in the room.

That nurse should be entertaining reasonable hunches of what might be going on and ruling them in or out—such as decreased oxygen saturation, increased pulmonary congestion, cardiac event, infectious process (such as pneumonia or urinary tract infection), medication side effect, or anxiety over the new environment. We'd expect that nurse to be considering his knowledge of such things as normal aging, for example, and that responses are usually blunted in elders. Other knowledge would be in such areas as typical heart failure signs, symptoms, and complications. We'd expect that nurse to communicate with the healthcare team about this event. We'd expect a nurse who has worked in that environment for several months to have some intuitive response to this situation, but not to jump to premature conclusions. Finally, we'd expect any nurse to take the situation seriously.

Some variations on this exercise would be to have staff or students discuss such scenarios in a group, have them write similar scenarios, and project what "wrong" things nurses might do in such situations.

PAUSE AND PONDER:
CONCLUSIONS ABOUT WHAT CT IS

This chapter was necessary to set the stage. Now, when someone asks you about CT, we hope you will have something more to say than, "That's a good question!" Understanding the concept of critical thinking is essential to nursing practice, but the ideas and words that describe the concept are only building blocks. Now we need to use those building blocks to nurture and expand CT in nursing. The next chapters will help you continue this life-long journey.

Reflection Cues

- CT bridges the gap between knowledge and actions.
- The Western history of CT can be traced as far back as Socrates to recent nursing research.

- CT in nursing is exemplified by 10 habits of the mind (*confidence, contextual perspective, creativity, flexibility, inquisitiveness, intellectual integrity, intuition, open-mindedness, perseverance, reflection*) and seven cognitive skills (*analyzing, applying standards, discriminating, information seeking, logical reasoning, predicting, transforming knowledge*).

- Dimensions of nursing CT not found in nonnursing descriptions are *creativity, intuition*, and *transforming knowledge*.

- Verbalizing one's CT requires descriptive language not commonly used in the action-oriented discipline of nursing.

- It is difficult to "see" the CT behind the actions. Actions must be combined with descriptions of thinking.

- Although most of us can identify colleagues who are good thinkers, it is very difficult to tease out the thinking behind their actions.

- Incorporating the language of thinking into our vocabulary increases our awareness of our own thinking, the thinking of others, and our ability to describe our thinking to colleagues.

References

American Association of Colleges of Nursing (AACN). (1998). *The essentials of baccalaureate education for professional nursing practice*. Washington, DC: Author.

American Nurses' Association (ANA). (2003). *Nursing: Scope and standards of practice*. Washington, DC: Author.

Benner, P. (1984). *From novice to expert: Power and excellence in nursing practice*. Menlo Park, CA: Addison-Wesley.

Case, B. (1998). Competence development: Critical thinking, clinical judgment, and technical ability. In K. J. Kelly-Thomas (Ed.), *Clinical & nursing staff development: Current competence, future focus* (pp. 240–281). Philadelphia: Lippincott.

Commission on Collegiate Nursing Education (CCNE). (2003). *Standards for accreditation of baccalaureate and graduate nursing programs*. Washington, DC: Author.

Costa, A. L. (Ed.) (1985). *Developing minds: A resource book for teaching thinking*. Alexandria, VA: Association for Supervision and Curriculum Development.

Dreyfus, H. L. & Dreyfus, S. E. (1986). *Mind over machine: The power of human intuition and expertise in the era of the computer*. New York: The Free Press.

Facione, P. A. (1990). *Critical thinking: A statement of expert consensus for purposes of educational assessment and instruction*. Millbrae, CA: The California Academic Press. (ERIC Document Reproduction Service No. ED315423)

Facione, N. C., Facione, P. A., & Sanchez, C. A. (1994). Critical thinking disposition as a measure of competent clinical judgment: The development of the California Critical Thinking Disposition Inventory. *Journal of Nursing Education, 33*(8), 345–350.

Facione, P. A., Sanchez, C. A., Facione, N. C., & Gainen, J. (1995). The disposition toward critical thinking. *Journal of Nursing Education, 44*(1), 1–25.

Fonteyn, M. E. (1998). *Thinking strategies for nursing practice.* Philadelphia: Lippincott.

Goodman, C. N. (1987). The Delphi technique: A critique. *Journal of Advanced Nursing, 12,* 729–734.

Hansten, R. I. & Washburn, M. J. (1999). Individual and organizational accountability for development of critical thinking. *Journal of Nursing Administration, 29*(11), 39–45.

Hart, L. A. (1983). *Human brain and human learning.* New York: Longman.

The Higher Learning Commission. (2003). Retrieved August 3, 2004, from http://www. ncacihe.org/overview/2003overview.pdf.

Institute of Medicine (IOM). (2004). *Keeping patients safe: Transforming the work environment for nurses.* Washington, DC: The National Academies Press.

Joint Commission on Accreditation of Healthcare Organizations (JCAHO). (2000). *Comprehensive accreditation manual for hospitals: The official handbook.* Chicago: Author.

Kant, I. (1965). *Critique of pure reason* (N. K. Smith, Trans.). New York: St. Martin's Press. (Original work published 1787)

Kemerling, G. (2002). *History of western philosophy.* Retrieved October 16, 2003, from http://www.philosophypages.com/hy/index.htm.

Miller, J., Galloway, M., Coughlin, C., & Brennan, E. (2001). Care-centered organizations, Part 1: Governance. *Journal of Nursing Administration, 31*(2), 67–73.

National League for Nursing Accrediting Commission (NLN-AC). (2003). *Accreditation manual for postsecondary and higher degree programs in nursing: Interpretive guidelines by program type.* New York: Author.

Rubenfeld, M. G. & Scheffer, B. K. (1999). *Critical thinking in nursing: An interactive approach* (2nd ed.). Philadelphia: Lippincott.

Scheffer, B. K. & Rubenfeld, M. G. (2000). A consensus statement on critical thinking in nursing. *Journal of Nursing Education, 39,* 352–359.

Schoenly, L. (1998). Staff development programs: Strategic thinking applied. In K. J. Kelly-Thomas (Ed.), *Clinical & nursing staff development: Current competence, future focus* (pp. 192–212). Philadelphia: Lippincott.

Tanner, C. (1997). Spock would have been a terrible nurse (and other issues related to critical thinking in nursing). *Journal of Nursing Education, 36*(1), 3–4.

Thompson, D. N. & Burns, H. K. (2004). Public Policy: Work environment for nurses and the impact on protecting patients from healthcare errors. *Journal of Professional Nursing, 20*(3), 145–146.

CHAPTER 3

Who Are the Critical Thinkers?

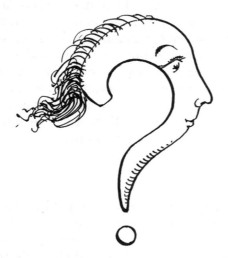

We have the *what* part of critical thinking (CT) figured out; now, *who* are the critical thinkers? Potentially everyone, but we're going to discuss people in healthcare practice and education settings because that's the focus of this book. And we're going to narrow our view even more to those of you who are reading these words.

Who are you? Most of you are probably nurses but, because these ideas are relevant to all healthcare providers, some of you may be from other disciplines. We hope so because, as we will discuss later, we are big believers in the necessity of interdisciplinary practice (see Chapter 7, in particular). Are you a clinician or an educator or does your position combine both roles? Perhaps you are a researcher, a manager, or an administrator in a practice setting. Nurses' roles and positions are often complex.

We needed to develop an organized way to address you that also fits with our proposed CT-enhancing tactics. As we see it, you readers want to improve your CT or help others improve theirs; therefore, we have decided to classify you as being in one of two categories—clinicians and educators. For clinicians, much of what we say will focus on how you can improve your CT; for educators, the focus will be on strategies to promote CT in others. We're aware that clinicians often try to help others improve CT and that educators should always work to improve their personal CT. Still, for ease of use the basic focus of self and others—that is clinicians and educators—will be used to address you, our readers, throughout this book.

A major reason why we've chosen to write to this audience is that we want to promote a unified view of CT as a vital, but complex, clinical and educational issue. We are quite aware that the literature on CT in nursing is primarily oriented toward those in academic settings—students and teachers. Indeed, most things we've written are academically slanted. However, the bottom line is that we all want to improve CT in clinical practice. If we don't start viewing this from both perspectives simultaneously we'll be building an ivory tower version and a digging-out-a-trench version. Neither will be adequate to meet the thinking demands of healthcare today or tomorrow.

CLINICIANS

We envision clinicians in a variety of healthcare settings. Many challenges tax your thinking skills, not the least of which is the seemingly constant change in the demands and responsibilities of your positions. Complex changes are occurring in healthcare delivery as a whole. Kelly-Thomas (1998) referred to the "re-do" words typically heard in healthcare environments these days—reengineering, restructuring, retooling, re-visioning. These re-do issues require, above all else, nurses to be confident, contextual, creative, open-minded, and flexible in their thinking strategies. We will return often to the subject of complex change, but especially in Chapter 11 where we discuss the realities of thinking yesterday, today, and tomorrow.

EDUCATORS

We envision educators in various settings as well, primarily as service-based (staff development specialists, continuing education directors, and so on) or academic-based (nursing school faculty). We expect that some of our clinicians and educators are graduate students pursuing one or both of those roles. Whichever kind of educator you are, you deal with many complex problems that affect how you see yourself as a thinker and how you'll be able to promote CT in your students and staff. Academic-based educators may be more familiar with CT language because much of what has been written about CT has been for traditional educational settings. We hope you will find this book to be helpful because it presents a practical view of CT, not just an academic view.

OTHER THINKERS WHO INTERACT WITH CLINICIANS AND EDUCATORS

Although for this discussion we've delineated two *who* groups and acknowledged that all people are thinkers, here is an important point: No one of us thinks in isolation. To view CT as an individual process will take us down a disastrous path where we waste time and money and, possibly, do harm. Other thinkers must also be considered, including patients, their significant others, and additional members of the healthcare team. We will address patient thinking in Chapter 6, and team thinking in Chapter 7, but, for now, remember that everything we say about CT applies to all the thinkers around you—other nurses, students, healthcare providers, patients and their significant others, administrators, politicians, and many others, to name only a few.

SELECTED FACTORS THAT AFFECT CRITICAL THINKERS

Many factors influence us as thinkers. For example, clinicians may be viewed as facing enormous challenges because their work is traditionally action oriented, taking place in settings that rarely sanction thinking time. Educators, on the other hand, are usually viewed as actively working when they sit with furrowed brows. In addition to these environmental factors, many other things influence one's thinking—genetics; self-concept; anxiety and other emotions; and culture, including family and cultural heritage, society, and organizational culture.

Genetics as an Influence on CT

Let's look at genetics, or basic "wiring," first. No two people think in the same way. (That's great, isn't it?) Whether those differences stem from genetics or one's upbringing is frequently debated. In reality it's both, but we do know that some differences are inborn. Some people have the ability to remember numerous esoteric facts but can't figure out how to solve simple everyday problems. Others never seem flustered when things go wrong, but can't remember when they last went to the bathroom. Acknowledging differences in thinking without judging that one way is better than another is a challenge, but a necessary one, especially for educators trying to individualize teaching strategies.

If you haven't thought about your natural, inborn thinking abilities, do that now. Refer to the short inventory in Box 2.4 on page 21 or the CT Inventory in Appendix A to help you reflect on this. If you can articulate your personal hard wiring it will make you a better learner. Are you a visual thinker? (You need to see it to understand it.) Are you an auditory thinker? (Once you hear it you remember it.) Do you have to do something with information, perform an action, before it stays in your brain? If you can describe to a teacher what works best for you, you will be a better learner. You will also be more sensitive to the learning and thinking styles of others and, therefore, be a better educator.

Consider this example from an author/educator: "My son has attention deficit disorder and, although his intelligence test results showed him to be above average, he could not learn how to add columns of numbers. When given a fourth-grade assignment to copy a list of numbers and add them, he would write the numbers in what seemed to be a random pattern so the tens or hundreds were never above and below each other. I kept saying to him, 'Line them up!' and he would repeatedly do this random thing. Finally, in total frustration, I drew lines on the sheet of paper. Then he had no trouble at all. It made me realize that he has no patterning ability in his mind remotely close to what I have in mine. Once we moved to graph paper with big squares, he was fine with addition of long sets of numbers." (By the way, this boy moved to the advanced math classes in high school.)

This example, in addition to illustrating vastly different thinking styles, also shows us that intelligence is not a simple construct. Howard Gardner deftly illustrated thinking complexity in his description of multiple intelligences (Gardner, 1983, 1993, 1999). Refer to Gardner's list in Box 3.1. Can you relate to some of those intelligences more than others? We'd guess yes. Gardner believed that we have varying proportions of each of these intelligences but that some of them come more naturally to us than others. That may be due to genetics and/or because some groups and cultures value some traits over others. Our self-concept of our thinking style is largely based on our dominant intelligences.

Self-Concept as an Influence on CT

Think about this statement: I am a great thinker. Do you believe it? If yes, why? If no, why? You can probably imagine a philosophy professor saying it. That's because we traditionally associate "great thinking" with fields such as philosophy. Nursing is traditionally associated with doing and actions. Both of these traditional associations are too limited, especially the nursing one. Expert nursing care requires expert levels of thinking for actions to be safe.

Obviously culture influences self-concept, but there's more to it than that, such as life circumstances and how much positive (or negative) feedback you get for your thinking ability. If your 10th grade math teacher told you, girls are never any good at math (and yes, teachers still say such things), the girls in that class would need some other equally dramatic evaluation of their math

---

Box 3.1

Gardner's Multiple Intelligences
(*Gardner, 1983; ~ Gardner, 1999)

- *Visual/Spatial:* the mind's eye: preference for use of images, pictures, graphical representations
- *Logical/Mathematical:* use of an entire range of reasoning skills, preference for factual data, and both inductive and deductive reasoning
- *Verbal/Linguistic:* embracing speaking and listening, reading, writing, and other forms of communication
- *Musical/Rhythmic:* patterned rhythms of the mind, learning and knowing by sharing, expressing, perceiving, and creating pitch and patterns
- *Bodily/Kinesthetic:* using the body as a conduit for the mind, using action and motion
- *Interpersonal/Social:* using the give and take of communication with intonation and punctuation with a goal of understanding, empathy, and learning from one another
- *Interpersonal/Introspective:* focusing on knowing self with a goal of internalizing learning through thoughtful connections and transformation of knowledge into meaning
- ~*Naturalist:* the ability to recognize and differentiate characteristics and phenomena of the plant and animal world as well as inorganic material
- ~*Spiritual:* concern with cosmic or existential issues; achievement of a state of being; and effect on others
- ~*Existential:* capacity to locate oneself with respect to the furthest reaches of the cosmos—the infinite and the infinitesimal—and the related capacity to locate oneself with respect to such existential features of the human condition as the significance of life, the meaning of death, the ultimate fate of the physical and the psychological worlds, and such profound experiences as love of another person or total immersion in a work of art.

skills to counter that attitude and develop a positive concept of themselves as mathematical thinkers. If you were always praised for your problem-solving abilities, you'd be proud of your analytical skills, promoting a positive self-concept in that CT dimension.

This example speaks to a very important point about the differences in how women and men think. Women and men are socialized differently, especially relative to self-concept and thinking ability. This is not an all-or-nothing interpretation, however. Excellent research has been done on female thinking (Gilligan, 1982, and Belenky, Clinchy, Goldberger & Tarule, 1986) and there are many helpful suggestions for addressing gender differences in classrooms (Brookfield & Preskill, 1999). Though gender has a significant influence on self-concept, and definitely is a force to be reckoned with in nursing with its lopsided ratio of women to men, even the experts caution us not to assume that gender is the only factor affecting how we think.

Unfortunately, women are still trying to escape the negative connotations of descriptions like "she's really smart," which cause most of us to flash back to high school where that meant, "she's not pretty." The implication there was that looks were more important than brains. Think of how women are described in the media even today; then consider how men are described—inevitably, women are described in terms of appearance and men are described in terms of intelligence or accomplishments.

While women have quite a few stereotypes working against them, men in nursing don't fare much better in how society views their thinking abilities. Because these men are nurses, not, for example, engineers, their thinking is considered less sophisticated. Unfortunately, people often judge a nontraditional career decision negatively, especially with respect to thinking ability. Why would a man do that (when he could have been an engineer or doctor)?

So the world doesn't view us as great thinkers and sees us through gender-biased eyes. Let's stop buying into those notions and work on what we do have control over—our self-concept as great thinkers. Simply reflecting on your thinking can help you improve your self-concept. After completing such reflection assignments, our students have said, "We never thought about our thinking before. We really *do* think a lot, don't we?" If we accept the stereotypical beliefs that we're not great thinkers, is it any wonder that we have self-concept problems about our thinking?

We need to value our brains and define ourselves as knowledge workers, not production workers. Kaeding and Rambur (2004) described knowledge work as "based on assessment, judgment, problem-solving, and the generation of ideas. It is nonrepetitive, nonroutine, and dependent on cognitive activity. Manual work is integral but not dominant. Gender is valued equally. Profes-

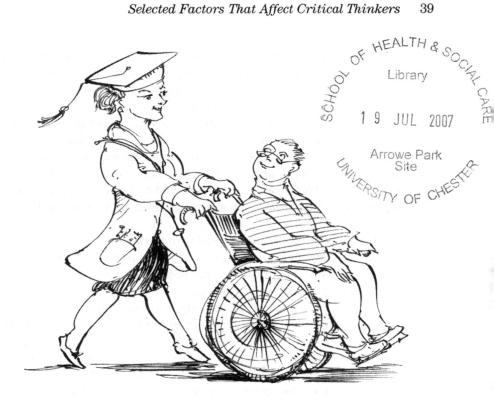

sional knowledge is not hierarchical, and evidence of learning is important to safe and effective job performance" (p. 137). Maybe we should go back to wearing nursing caps, but this time we should make them in the shape of mortar-boards representing the knowledge gleaned through education and experience.

Feelings, Especially Anxiety, As Influences on CT

Another major factor that influences thinking involves emotions. Intense feelings of love, hate, depression, elation—will always be factors shaping our cognitive skills. When we did our Delphi study to find consensus on CT, we specifically asked about habits of the mind in addition to cognitive skills. Most people, at least in nursing, acknowledge that CT has both affective (habits of the mind) and cognitive (skills) components. Those two components exist in tandem all the time. But, when we add an extreme emotional response to a situation, affective components of CT exert a stronger influence.

Many mood states affect thinking, but anxiety is particularly important in the healthcare sector, which has more than its share of anxiety-producing situations. Most older nurses (age 50 or above) can tell horror stories about how they were so terrified by nursing school teachers that they couldn't think at all. Hart (1983) called that "reptilian" brain functioning meaning the higher-order thinking skills of mammals shuts down and only basic survival thinking takes over. Teaching through terror, we hope, has gone the way of our nursing caps. Nevertheless, doing a nursing task for the first time, even with a nurturing teacher to help, still makes our hearts race and our palms dampen. And some nursing tasks continue to make us anxious even after we've done them many times.

Many self-help books on how to deal with anxiety exist, so we're not going to give a short course here. However, we do encourage all of you to consider what happens to your thinking when you're anxious and what circumstances, in particular, make you anxious. Also, consider what Margaret Carson (2003) called the "emotional burden" of nursing. Carson studied nurses who had been in combat situations, but she also cautioned nurses to consider the psychological toll of other high-stress nursing situations. In our experience nurses do not do a good job of taking care of themselves; we need to think about our emotional responses more, value things like lunch and bathroom breaks, and consider the importance of decreasing anxiety to sharpen our thinking skills.

If you teach others, orient new staff, or function as a preceptor we have a special message for you: If you expect your students and staff to be good thinkers, you must guide them gently, acknowledge their anxiety, and employ teaching and mentoring strategies, such as humor, that reduce anxiety. It is both humbling and helpful to remember your first lecture or your first attempt to catheterize an uncooperative patient. Telling students about your fears or relating to new staff how you botched simple jobs in your first weeks on the unit can do wonders to help them relax and reassure them they will also gain mastery. Most of all, we must approach teaching as a collaborative effort, not a game of one-upmanship, where you are the all-knowing expert and your students have blank slates for brains. Anxiety is a day-to-day reality of nursing. We need to acknowledge it, remember its influence on thinking, and constantly work to lessen it, to help ourselves and others.

Cultural Influences on CT

Unquestionably, we are influenced by our native culture and by the culture in which we live and work. Depending on your level of ethnocentrism or your exposure to different cultures, you may not realize how deeply cultural norms affect your thinking and that of people around you.

Culture, as defined by Giger and Davidhizar (2004), is:

> a patterned behavioral response that develops over time as a result of imprinting the mind through social and religious structures and intellectual and artistic manifestations. Culture is also the result of acquired mechanisms that may have innate influences but are primarily affected by internal and external environmental stimuli. Culture is shaped by values, beliefs, norms, and practices that are shared by members of the same cultural group. Culture guides our thinking, doing, and being and becomes patterned expressions of who we are (p. 3).

Culture is not static; it changes with time as cultural groups change definitions of their parameters. Although we can trace almost everything we think and do back to some cultural influence, there are some aspects of culture that are especially relevant when it comes to CT, particularly communication and time orientation. We will also discuss the organizational culture of the health-care work environment and how it affects CT.

Communication, Culture, and CT

Communication is the most obvious area where culture could affect CT. The term communication covers a broad range of topics about which numerous books are written. In this section, we focus on two: language and translation of meaning across cultures, and one's style for communicating thinking.

First, consider what language a person speaks. Is it the language of the majority? If not, consider what implications translation can have on the various components of CT. Words to describe thinking are complex, abstract, and often have no direct translation in other languages. On a recent trip to Japan to present a paper on CT, we found that the phrase, *habits of the mind*, caused the most complex translation problem. There was no direct translation so we tried to think of a synonym. Remember that we chose that phrase deliberately because we wanted to get across these finer points: The word *traits* often connotes static qualities, and we wanted to stay away from that. *Characteristics* was too broad; *dispositions* was closely aligned with traits. As the translator tried these and other words, she became very frustrated. *Tendencies toward* seemed to work as did *affinity for*, but ultimately the complete meaning of habits of the mind was probably never effectively translated.

What did this do to our discussion about CT? In this case, the idea that habits of the mind can be enhanced and our suggestions on how to do that may literally have gotten lost in translation. Because language is the basis of understanding, the very words used to describe CT and its dimensions need to be clarified at the outset of any discussion. If we aren't using the same descriptors, we may not be talking about the same thing.

Second, consider the different styles of communication that exist among cultural groups. As we stated in Chapter 2, CT requires questioning, but how is questioning viewed in other cultures? Is it considered an impolite or a desirable activity? Group activities to enhance CT usually involve sharing thoughts about thinking style; such sharing can be seen as a very intimate process. Do some cultures have "rules" prohibiting such personal exchanges?

I (Gaie) will switch to singular first-person writing here for a moment because this observation is personal. I can think of two extremes to illustrate the differences in communication style among cultures. One occurred in my native Newfoundland, a small maritime province in Canada. The other occurred in Japan, where I recently did the presentation on CT to which I referred earlier. I have not lived in Newfoundland for many years, but I visit frequently. It seems that there is open debate on everything in my home province. I have never seen a place with so many radio talk shows! Everyone has an opinion on everything and they freely express it through whatever medium is available. Several people talking at once, using emphatic gestures, is more the norm than the exception. While doing a presentation on CT to nurses there several years ago, I had to stop frequently for discussion and questions from the audience. To someone unfamiliar with the culture, the questions might have seemed confrontational. I felt right at home!

In Japan, on the other hand, the large audience of nurses was extremely quiet. I was a bit intimidated when I walked into the auditorium to find 3,000 nurses who were so silent it reminded me of how the room sounded the day before while I rehearsed—but then it was completely empty. I'm used to the din that American and Canadian audiences make as they wait for programs to begin. In Japan, when I asked for questions, there were few. Those who spoke did not use hand gestures and began each interaction with a deferential comment, such as "excuse me." Japanese nursing faculty, who are very interested in promoting CT, told me they have to repeatedly encourage students to discuss issues and ask questions; students there are much more comfortable with lectures.

Extremes such as these, and all kinds of examples in between, occur in nursing practice and schools throughout North America as well. What do such differences mean to the educator or clinician? Because questioning is considered a desirable part of CT, the tendency is to believe that the assertive communicator is a better critical thinker. However, we must consider just what it is that we most value. Is it the communication of questions or the questioning itself that is important? Perhaps we need to think of ways beyond verbal means to encourage questioning. Perhaps quiet people are more comfortable sharing their questions in writing. Smaller group discussions that are not teacher led or web caucuses might be more appropriate for those from cultures where open questioning is seen as impolite.

Time Orientation, Culture, and CT

If communication styles seem culturally bound, what about other things such as the cultural influence on time orientation? There is a certain expectation of a "futuristic view" in nursing descriptions of CT. Speaking generally, certain groups have one of three dominant time perspectives—past, present, or future. Of course, there are many exceptions to these broad generalizations, but we usually view Eastern cultures as more focused on the past, Hispanic and Native American/Aboriginal cultures as more focused on the present, and European–American cultures as more focused on the future.

A Hispanic nurse once told us that he asks Hispanic patients if they'd like him to record appointment times on their cards half an hour earlier so they'd be on time for their appointments. He initiates that question with a comment about his own tendency for tardiness because he's not very future oriented.

Another example from Gaie: a friend and I recently stopped to visit a basket maker on a Mi'kmaq reservation in Cape Breton, Nova Scotia. We were so fascinated with her exquisite weaving of a quill basket, we stayed longer than planned. Upon realizing the time we jumped up, saying, "We'll be late getting to our friend's house. We need to get going." The basket maker looked at us, smiled, and said, "Just tell them you were on the res' and you're on Indian time." Clearly, her present-oriented perspective was so much a part of her culture that she was very comfortable making humorous references to it. Later I thought about what it would be like if she were a student in my CT class. What would she think when I stressed the importance of "predicting" (one of the CT skills we identified in our study) as part of CT? Would she adopt a futuristic thinking mode because it was expected? How would that affect other parts of her thinking, honed by years of her own culture's influence?

Another issue relative to time is the predominant US value of time-is-money. Along with time-is-money comes time-equals-action. For vivid examples of this in healthcare, we only have to look at managed care approaches where nurse practitioners and physicians are required to see large numbers of patients each hour to meet income quotas. Home healthcare nurses are given similar quota directives—ones that make quality care difficult. What happens to CT in a culture that clearly values the tangible results of work, but not the process of improving quality through thinking? It takes time to think; some things take longer to think about than others; and some people think faster or slower than others.

Box 3.2

Cultural Influences on Thinking Habits of the Mind

Directions: Place an X on the line to indicate your self-rating.

My culture:

values   encourages
limited   open
questioning   debate
of authority _____   for all.

is primarily focused on the
    past _____ present _____ future _____

values contemplation _____ values actions _____

In my culture I am encouraged to:

be confident of my reasoning ability
            never _____ always

consider where someone is coming from when I interact
            never _____ always

be as creative as possible
            never _____ always

be flexible, even if it means changing my expectations
            never _____ always

be openly inquisitive
            never _____ always

seek the truth, even if it differs from my beliefs
            never _____ always

be sensitive to my gut feelings
            never _____ always

reflect on my biases
            never _____ always

stick to something until I accomplish it
            never _____ always

spend time reflecting on my thinking and actions
            never _____ always

TACTICS 3.1: Cultural Influences on Thinkers

Clinician

Using the checklist in Box 3.2, reflect on your culture and how it might affect your CT habits of the mind. Then think of someone you work with who comes from a different culture than yours. Think of a patient from a different culture. How do you think those persons would answer the questions?

Educators

Use the checklist in Box 3.2, as the basis for a group discussion. Consider whether your students and staff gain an awareness of other cultures.

Discussion

Did you learn anything about your culture? Other people's cultures? You've probably considered such things before, but have you put them into a CT frame of reference? We tend to think of cultural norms in terms of such things as eating, holidays, dress, but we don't often associate them with our thinking.

Organizational Culture and CT

This brings us to a significant cultural influence on you as a thinker—the organizational culture of your work environment. We discuss organizational cultures more in Chapter 5 under *how, when, and where* to think, and again in Chapter 11 when we discuss day-to-day realities; here we consider how much your employment environment defines you as a thinker. Much has been written about the influence of work environment on thinking (e.g., Senge, 1990; Chan, 2001). In her study of nursing preceptorship, Myrick (2002) identified the work climate or environment as a key variable enabling CT.

Organizational cultures can be very powerful. There is a strong tendency to assume that behaving in accordance with one's organizational culture is the "correct" way to do things and avoids role conflict. Such assumptions generally lead to a status quo environment that precludes thinking. After all, it's easy. Status quo thinking, however, is not healthy and eventually leads to the decline, entropy, and ultimate demise of the organization (Higgins, 1995).

Organizational cultures that promote a status quo existence are potentially dangerous to critical thinkers. Brookfield (1993) recognized this situation and warned critically thinking nurses about "cultural suicide" (being ostracized by coworkers as a result of challenging the status quo). Many critically thinking nurses are thought of as being on the fringes of mainstream thinking because they question, challenge, and annoy those who prefer to keep things the same.

Although few would admit to this, today's complex systems of healthcare practice and education often blatantly discourage CT. Mohr, Deatrick, Richmond and Mahon (2001) addressed organizational values conflicts, painting a picture of troubled organizations. Some unhealthy traits they mentioned: overcontrol, distraction with minutiae, repression, intolerance for new members and diversity, territorial behaviors, depression, submissiveness, and horizontal violence (passive–aggressive behavior). This is a culture that will certainly not contribute to the growth of its members' CT.

Organizational cultures that encourage CT and acknowledge the inevitability of change are called "learning organizations" and they use "systems thinking" (Senge, 1990; Chan, 2001). Their members exhibit traits of trustworthiness, autonomy, responsibility, and reflection (Mohr et al., 2001). They rely on resources such as books, computers, links to libraries, and librarians. They provide think time and emphasize language/description and sharing of thinking. They give verbal "credit" and reward the thinking process, not just the end product. They welcome debate. If you are fortunate enough to work in that kind of environment, it is bound to positively influence you as a thinker. People like us, who spend a lot of time thinking about thinking, define such places as heaven, nirvana; we dream about such organizational cultures and hope to see them as the norm in nursing.

TACTICS 3.2: Environmental Factors Influencing Thinkers

Clinicians

Think about your environment. Generally speaking:
1. Where does it fall on the continuum from status quo thinking to our description of thinking heaven?
2. What is your position in that environment?
3. Can you influence the working culture?
4. How could you influence it?
5. Make a list of things you can influence in your environment that would make it more thinking-friendly.

Educators

Think about your teaching style.
1. Complete the checklist in Box 3.3.
2. How would you rate yourself as a positive influence on the thinking of your learners?
3. Review one of your teaching plans; do you see evidence of thinking-promoting strategies?
4. Can you or should you change anything in your plan?

Discussion

How does your environmental culture stack up? Are you doing a good job of promoting CT in your organization? Cultures that promote critical

---

Box 3.3

Thinking-Promoting Teaching Style Checklist

In my teaching I:
- evaluate and give credit for thinking processes (e.g., "good thinking!").
- use multisensory techniques.
- encourage lots of questions.
- do not get defensive when questioned or challenged.
- help students find information resources.
- describe to students how I think, model my thinking.
- use deliberate methods to decrease anxiety.
- develop teaching objectives/expected competencies that go beyond recall of information and require transforming information into usable knowledge.
- use humor.
- create a thinking-friendly environmental culture that accepts "mistakes" as opportunities to grow.
- vary teaching methods and strategies throughout each session.
- engage students in peer review activities.
- provide written reflection time in class.
- ask students to expand on their answers (e.g., "Tell me more").
- promote students' positive self-concepts.
- emphasize collaborative learning between teacher and student (as opposed to authoritarian style).
- allow/encourage the student to be the teacher.

---

thinking have members who think individually and collectively. Such organizations are not neat; indeed they appear rather chaotic. They are in a constant state of change. We'll discuss this change process in Chapter 11, but for now think about what kind of thinker you are and how much that part of you is defined by your work culture. What can you do to make your environment more conducive to CT?

This reflection process helps to identify who in your organization are potential critical thinking mentors. Not all members of an organization strive to be great thinkers. The larger the numbers of critical thinkers in an organization, the better the quality of healthcare.

PAUSE AND PONDER:
DEFINING OURSELVES AS CRITICAL THINKERS

In this chapter we have focused on clinicians and educators who are the keys to promoting CT in nursing. Once again, let us caution you: CT is not just an individual phenomena. Our CT is influenced by all of the thinkers around us and we influence their thinking, too. Repeatedly throughout this book we assert the importance of this point. Today's healthcare delivery and educational systems are enormously complex. If clinicians and educators don't define themselves as critical thinkers, we will have enormous problems.

Reflection Cues

- This chapter specifically speaks to clinicians and educators about their identities as thinkers.
- Many factors influence one's development as a critical thinker.
- Genetics or one's natural thinking processes influence who you are as a thinker.
- Gardner's multiple intelligences increase our awareness of different styles of thinking and processing information.
- Self-concept as an influence on CT is shaped by many factors such as gender and social mores.
- Nurses are great thinkers, even though the world doesn't always see them as such or acknowledge their thinking as essential to their actions.
- Nurses are knowledge workers, not production workers.
- All emotions, but especially anxiety, exert a huge influence on one's CT.
- Both our native cultures and the cultures in which we live and work influence us as thinkers.
- Cultural differences in communication and time orientation affect who we become as thinkers.
- Organizational cultures can help or hinder one's development as a thinker.
- Cultures that discourage CT have traits such as intolerance, territorial behaviors, and repression.

- Organizational cultures that promote CT are called learning environments and use more systems thinking.
- We need to reflect on who we are as thinkers and how we promote a culture of thinking.
- Clinicians and educators must promote a unified view of CT as being vital to both practice and educational settings.

References

Belenky, M. F., Clinchy, B. M., Goldberger, N. R., & Tarule, J. M. (1986). *Women's ways of knowing: The development of self, voice, and mind.* New York: Basic Books.

Brookfield, S. (1993). On impostorship, cultural suicide, and other dangers: How nurses learn critical thinking. *The Journal of Continuing Education in Nursing, 24*(5), 197–205.

Brookfield, S. D. & Preskill, S. (1999). *Discussion as a way of teaching: Tools and techniques for democratic classrooms.* San Francisco: Jossey-Bass.

Carson, M. (2003, November). *There to Care: A Lesson From Nursing History.* Paper presented at the 37th Biennial Convention of Sigma Theta Tau International, Toronto, Ontario, Canada.

Chan, C-P. C. A. (2001). Implications of organizational learning for nursing managers from the cultural, interpersonal and systems thinking perspectives. *Nursing Inquiry, 8,* 196–199.

Gardner, H. (1983). *Frames of mind: The theory of multiple intelligences* (10th anniversary ed.). New York: Basic Books.

Gardner, H. (1993). *Multiple intelligences: The theory in practice.* New York: Basic Books.

Gardner, H. (1999). *Intelligence reframed: Multiple intelligences for the 21st century.* New York: Basic Books.

Giger, J. N. & Davidhizar, R. E. (2004). *Transcultural nursing: Assessment and intervention* (4th ed.). St. Louis: Mosby.

Gilligan, C. (1982). *In a different voice: Psychological theory and women's development.* Cambridge, MA: Harvard University Press.

Hart, L. A. (1983). *Human brain and human learning.* New York: Longman.

Higgins, J. M. (1995). Innovate or evaporate: Seven secrets of innovative corporations. *The Futurist, 29*(5), 42–48.

Kaeding, T. H. & Rambur, B. (2004). Recruiting knowledge, not just nurses. *Journal of Professional Nursing, 20*(2), 137–138.

Kelly-Thomas, K. J. (1998). *Clinical and nursing staff development: Current competence, future focus* (2nd ed.). Philadelphia: Lippincott.

Mohr, W. K., Deatrick, J., Richmond, T., & Mahon, M. M. (2001). A reflection on values in turbulent times. *Nursing Outlook, 49,* 30–36.

Myrick, F. (2002). Preceptorship and critical thinking in nursing education. *Journal of Nursing Education, 41*(4), 154–164.

Senge, P. M. (1990). *The fifth discipline: The art & practice of the learning organization.* New York: Doubleday.

CHAPTER 4

Why Is Critical Thinking So Important?

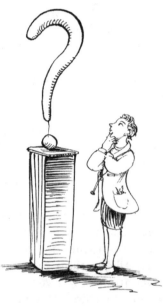

Now wait a minute! I've done colostomy dressing changes a dozen times, I followed all the steps of the protocol exactly as I always do. Afterward I even checked out the textbook the nursing student left on the unit and it says to do exactly what I did. So I'm asking myself, why didn't it work? (Joyce, novice clinician)

This critical thinking (CT) reflection occurred at an early stage of Joyce's attempts to understand why her intervention did not work. The inquisitive clinician, student, or educator begins many thinking journeys with the word *why*? We'll get back to Joyce's thinking later in this chapter. *Why* is the next logical phase of inquiry after *what* and *who*. Specifically, *why* is CT so important? We have devoted a whole chapter to answering this because it clarifies the value of CT and provides justification for all the hard work that CT requires. First, we will examine the importance of *why* questions and take a look at *why* the attention paid to CT has grown over the last two decades. We will look at the bigger picture of *why* CT is so important to each stakeholder in healthcare. And finally, we'll explore *why* we need to talk about CT more.

WHY QUESTIONS AND THINKING

Why questions imply a search for reason, purpose, meaning, and value. Let's look at reason first. The word *why* is frequently used to initiate inquiry, provide logic, justify conclusions, and find causes. In Joyce's situation, she wanted to know *why* the dressing fell off.

Why demonstrates one of the first forms of thinking and exploration we used as children ("Why is the sky blue?"). Those of you with young children who constantly ask *why*, might want the word banned from the dictionary. But *why* and the thinking connected with *why* have triggered many important discoveries over the years. The discovery of penicillin, Einstein's Theory of Relativity, the exploration of space, and even the discovery of Viagra all followed *why*. (In fact, according to a personal communication with a pharmaceutical industry research scientist, it was a nurse who asked the question that led to the discovery of Viagra as a treatment for erectile dysfunction. During clinical trials of a pharmacological treatment of cardiovascular problems, she noticed that the volunteers were reluctant to return unused trial medications. She asked *why*, and the rest is history!)

For many, the natural tendency to ask *why* has diminished after years of traditional schooling. That is sad and also a bit frightening because *why* questions are powerful instigators of thinking. Remember the CT inventory in Chapter 2 and Appendix A? All questions related to *information seeking* and *inquisitiveness* are derived from *why*. Even Albert Einstein emphasized the value of *why* questions when he said: "The important thing is to never stop questioning. Curiosity has its own reason for existing," and "I am neither especially clever nor gifted, I am only very very curious" ("Famous Quotes," n.d.).

Why is also the favorite word of many educators who encourage students to provide rationales for their nursing interventions. *Why* is used by clinicians when they work as preceptors and mentors for new staff or when they question their own practice, as Joyce did earlier. Clinicians and educators alike believe *why* questions encourage critical thinking (Scheffer, 2001).

TACTICS 4.1: Exploring Your Use of *Why*

Clinicians and Educators

With a colleague or on your own, think about the last time you asked *why*? How many times a day do you ask it? Enough times to learn what you want to know? Too many? And what does it lead to? Are you simply asking out of habit or do you then pursue the answers that then prompt you to ask more questions and delve even deeper? How do colleagues react to your *why* questions? What motivates you to ask *why*?

Discussion

The answers to these questions should stimulate reflection. Are you satisfied with your answers? We believe the number of *why* questions you ask correlates highly with your CT dimensions of *information seeking, inquisitiveness,* and *reflection.*

Why questions that stimulate *reflection* can prompt searches for purpose, meaning, and value. The great philosophers asked all of these classic questions: *Why* are we here? *Why* do we exist? *Why* do we care? On a less esoteric level, *reflection* on *why* helps us understand and appreciate the value of thinking. So *why* does CT benefit healthcare? To answer, we will look at *why* there has been so much interest in thinking in recent years. We will also respond to *why* thinking is so important.

WHY THE GROWING INTEREST IN CT?

As described in Chapter 2, thinking has been a topic of discussion for philosophers for centuries, but other disciplines have also been concerned about thinking. Schon (1983) cited examination of thinking in medicine, engineering, law, business, and education. Dreyfus and Dreyfus (1986) described the importance of thinking in the aviation industry.

There are hundreds of thousands of articles and thousands of books written about CT in all disciplines. There are courses, whole curricula, and even institutes designed to improve thinking. We taught a required undergraduate nursing course called, "Critical Thinking in Nursing" for several years. Alverno College in Madison, Wisconsin, has designed the mission, philosophy and all of its program curricula (including nursing) around reasoning, analysis, and reflection ("Alverno College, Academics, Nursing," 2004, para 10). There is even a consortium of institutes focused on critical thinking, which includes the Center for Critical Thinking, The National Council for Excellence in Critical Thinking, and the International Center for the Assessment of Higher Order Thinking ("Critical Thinking Consortium," 2004). An Australian website (http://www.austhink.org/critical/pages/institutes.html) provides up-to-date information on colleges, universities, forums, and ongoing research on CT ("Institutes, Centers and Societies, Nursing," 2004).

In healthcare, accrediting bodies, policy makers, and others promote CT. For example, the National League for Nursing Accrediting Commission (NLN-AC) included CT in its accreditation criteria (NLN-AC, 2003). The Institute of Medicine (IOM) (2004) addressed CT across disciplines for improving national healthcare. Obviously, many people and organizations think critical thinking is very important; some of their statements about the benefits of thinking are shown in Box 4.1.

So why has there been so much emphasis on CT in healthcare over the last few decades? One only has to pick up a newspaper or magazine or listen to the news to learn the answer. Some of the key matters that require more or better thinking are the information explosion; dwindling resources; cost containment; third-party payer gatekeeping; morbidity and mortality data; patient safety and failure to rescue; and emergent ethical dilemmas, such as the right to life, prolongation of life without quality, and stem cell research.

All healthcare disciplines are recognizing the need to pool their thinking to come up with ways to deal with such complex issues. A notable example of such pooled thinking is the IOM project (2003). The project's charge was to tap into the thinking energy of an interdisciplinary group—nurses, physicians, pharmacists, physical therapists, social workers, and others—to identify new directions for healthcare. Past solutions clearly do not address the growing complexity of our current problems. If it's not working today, it surely will fail tomorrow. To quote from Albert Einstein again, "The significant problems we face cannot be solved at the same level of thinking we were at when we created them" ("Famous Quotes," n.d.).

One outcome of the IOM work was the development of five competencies—*patient-centered care, interdisciplinary teams, evidence-based practice, informatics,* and *quality improvement* (2003). These competencies were developed to help guide the thinking of all healthcare disciplines toward a unified plan of practice, education, and research to promote safe, effective, and efficient patient care. We will discuss these competencies fully in Chapters 5 through 10, but for now, let's look at some of the basic benefits of thinking in healthcare and who benefits from it. We'll start by seeing if we can help Joyce, the novice clinician, who had trouble with the colostomy dressing.

TACTICS 4.2: Exploring Joyce's Thinking

Let's review Joyce's situation:

> Now wait a minute! I've done colostomy dressing changes a dozen times, I followed all the steps of the protocol exactly as I always do. Afterward I even checked out the textbook the nursing student left on the unit and it says to do exactly what I did. So I'm asking myself, why didn't it work?

Now refer to Box 4.1 and see if you can find any clues that would help Joyce. Then look at your list of CT habits of mind and skills in Chapter 2

Box 4.1

Statements About the Benefits of CT

"Professional knowledge is mismatched to the changing characteristics of the situation of practice—the complexity, uncertainty, instability, uniqueness, and value conflicts, which are increasingly perceived as central to the world of professional practice." (Schon, 1983, p. 14)

Problems encountered in practice are not in the book. (Schon, 1983)

"Knowledge is discovered by thinking, analyzed by thinking, organized by thinking, transformed by thinking, assessed by thinking, and most importantly acquired by thinking." (Paul, 1992, p. xi)

Thinking helps us recognize beliefs and assumptions that our minds consider to be facts. (Brookfield, 1995)

Knowledge, facts, and information are frequently equated with intelligence. But the ability to use knowledge in logical, ethical, and moral ways is not always equal to the quality of the knowledge, facts and information. Thinking provides the screening mechanism for converting knowledge, facts and information into practical application in the real world. (Schon, 1983)

"...no way to create a neat and tidy step-by-step path to knowledge that all minds can mindlessly follow." (Paul, 1992, p. xi)

Pure logic and analytical reasoning is inadequate for expert decision making. Expert decision making is a blend of careful analysis, intuition and the wisdom and judgment gleaned from experience. Human thinking and decision making continues to exceed that of machines (artificial intelligence) because of three key factors: awareness of the environment, the ability to discriminate, and tolerance for ambiguity. (Dreyfus & Dreyfus, 1986)

"Only by changing how we think can we change deeply embedded policies and practices." (Senge, 1990, p. xiv)

"the deepest insight usually comes when they [people] realize that their problems, and their hopes for improvement, are inextricably tied to how they think." (Senge, 1990, p. 53)

Self-regulation, critical thinking, and creative thinking are probably the most important dimensions influencing learning. (Marzano & Pickering, 1997)

True understanding comes from the ability to think and act flexibly, distinguish nuance, appreciate context, and use reflection. (Wiggins & McTighe, 2001) (or on your tear-out card) and identify which CT dimensions Joyce used. What others, had she used them, would have been beneficial?

Discussion

The second statement in Box 4.1, "Problems encountered in practice are not in the book" (Schon, 1983), is a good match for what happened to Joyce. Do other statements also fit? What about the 17 CT dimensions? Joyce did use: *applying standards*, when she used the protocols for colostomy dressing changes; *information seeking*, when she went to the textbook; the beginnings of *perseverance*, as she seemed to want to find an answer; and definitely *reflection*, as she wondered what went wrong. The dimensions of thinking that might have helped Joyce, but which she did not use are: *discrimination* (was there something about this patient's colostomy that differed from others she had changed in the past?); *contextual perspective* (was something about this patient's situation unique, such as his skin condition, the stoma site, the moisture around the stoma?); and *analysis* (did she break down all the aspects of the situation, the equipment used, effectiveness of the adhesive, the time of day, and so on?). Were you able to identify more?

This is a simple example of *why* CT is necessary in nursing and why we need to understand and use more than one CT dimension at a time. Nurses must be comfortable with and be able to use the constellation of 17 dimensions, in different combinations, or a host of other healthcare problems might arise.

The next section of this chapter explores the magnitude of thinking needed in nursing and healthcare. It focuses on the big picture of CT and the value thinking has to all stakeholders. It also addresses the complexity of thinking needed in the healthcare environment.

THE BIG PICTURE OF *WHY* THINKING IS IMPORTANT

We've learned that the purpose of asking *why* is to find meaning and value or benefit. To focus on benefits we need to explore who benefits and what is the benefit—*why* is thinking important to them? We will use the term "stakeholders" to describe these groups because it has a broad scope. Stakeholder is a term used in organizational literature to describe the groups who have a "stake" in some endeavor. Stakeholders gain or lose something, such as power, control, money, and—yes—health. They are also thinkers because they gain or lose from thinking or not thinking. And their thinking has an effect on the whole, as well. See how complex this is?

Clinicians and educators are only two groups in a whole galaxy of stakeholders. Figure 4.2 illustrates this metaphorical galaxy. We used an astronomy

Figure 4.2   Galaxy of Thinking Stakeholders

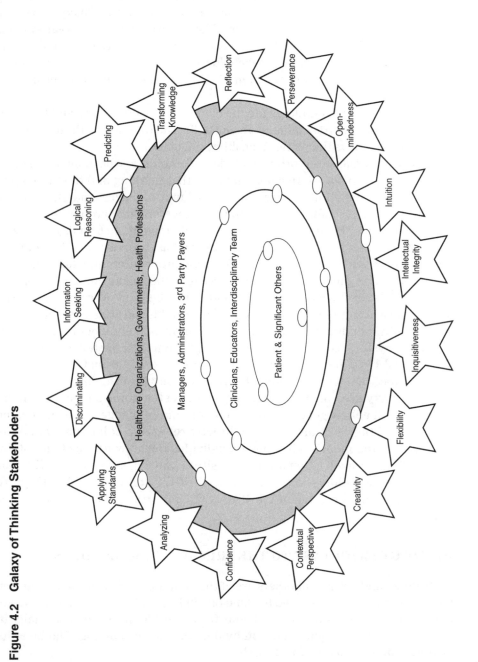

metaphor because it captures the dynamic nature of thinking and the vastness of CT needed in healthcare. Galaxies, just like healthcare systems, are very complex entities in constant flux. Change in one part of the galaxy, or healthcare system, affects all the other parts. Galaxies are made up of solar systems and the constellations of stars. In the healthcare system, patients and their significant others are the primary stakeholders (because they both participate in the thinking and directly benefit from it). They are the center of the healthcare galaxy.

The secondary stakeholders are the clinicians, the educators, and the other providers of the Interdisciplinary Team (IDT). The thinking of these "planets" most directly affects the patient's healthcare needs.

Two additional outer orbits include stakeholders who contribute their thinking, but who also derive benefits from that thinking and the thinking of others. These stakeholders are made up of unit managers, administrators, third-party payers, healthcare organizations, governmental groups, and healthcare professions. Their CT may have a less obvious impact on day-to-day issues of patient care, however, this impact has broader and longer-term consequences, such as legislation, policies and procedures, and guidelines.

In addition to the planets in the solar system, the galaxy contains a constellation of 17 "stars," which shine back and reflect light on everything else. The stars represent the 17 CT dimensions. When thinking is at its best, they shine very brightly, blindingly bright at times. All of the stakeholders in this healthcare solar system use the bright light energy from the constellation of stars. They use all 17 CT dimensions to derive the most benefit from CT.

The galaxy analogy highlights the dynamic nature of thinking: all the bodies in a galaxy are constantly moving, some faster, some slower. When objects in a real galaxy get close to each other, things change; for instance, the weather and the tides on earth are directly related to solar energy and the proximity of the moon. In healthcare, individuals who work together continually influence each other's CT in positive and negative ways. With our galaxy of stakeholders and constellation of CT stars in mind, let's more closely examine the value of CT. *Why* is CT important to each stakeholder group?

WHY IS CT IMPORTANT TO THE PRIMARY STAKEHOLDERS?

Patients and significant others are at the center of our healthcare solar system, but the 17 CT "stars" need to shine on all! Remember, too, that each stakeholder benefits from his own CT and from the CT of others, especially in healthcare, which requires both individual and team thinking. The benefits identified here are a function of both.

Why Is CT Important to Patients and Significant Others?

This is a bit of a no-brainer. In Chapter 10 we delve into CT and the delivery of safe, effective, and efficient care; for now we will simply say that these have always been the underlying goals of good nursing care. CT is essential to achieving these goals. (See Box 4.2.)

Box 4.2

Why Is CT Important to Patients and Significant Others?

Thinking promotes safe care.
Thinking enhances effective care.
Thinking increases efficient care.

The following TACTICS exercise highlights how nursing staff using—or not using—CT affects the primary stakeholder, the patient. This exercise could be used by clinicians or educators to emphasize why thinking is important to safe, effective, and efficient patient care.

TACTICS 4.3: Exploring Safe, Effective, and Efficient Care for Mr. Stone

1. Read the scenario about Mr. Stone.
2. As you read, think about which of the 17 CT dimensions were used in providing his care.
3. Identify which CT dimensions were probably not used.

Scenario 4.1

Mr. Stone

Mr. Stone is a 60-year-old male. He was admitted to the hospital three days before the Christmas holiday for emergency surgery after his left arm was severed midway between his wrist and elbow in an industrial accident. He was in good health prior to the accident but had smoked one to two packs of cigarettes a day for 40 years. The surgery to remove the severed portion of his arm and create a stump for a prosthesis was successful. Nursing care included administration of pain medications, monitoring for infection at the wound site, and assistance with activities of daily living. Mr. Stone was expected to be

*discharged in two to three days. On day two after surgery he devel-
oped pneumonia and his hospital stay was extended six more days.*

Discussion

What CT dimensions did you identify? The ones that *should* have been used, but probably were not, and which may have contributed to Mr. Stone's pneumonia, include: *applying standards, contextual perspective, discriminating,* and *predicting.* If the nurses were *applying standards*, they would have designed care to include coughing, incentive spirometry, and tight assessment of respiratory status when developing their post-op care plan, not just medications and wound care. If the nurses were using *contextual perspective*, they would have more carefully assessed Mr. Stone's smoking habits and any history of respiratory problems. If the nurses were *discriminating*, they would have identified Mr. Stone as a very high-risk patient for post-op pulmonary complications because of his smoking. If the nurses were *predicting*, they would have recognized the serious consequences of not developing a rigorous plan for post-op coughing and deep-breathing. They might even have made a referral to respiratory therapy to institute such a prevention plan.

Of course, Mr. Stone might have developed pneumonia in spite of all those nursing interventions; however with better critical thinking, the chances of this outcome would have been greatly reduced. Not only did Mr. Stone suffer the physical and emotional pain of loss of an arm and early retirement, but because of his potentially preventable pneumonia he was hospitalized over the Christmas and New Year's Day holidays, a favorite time of year he would have enjoyed with family and friends at home.

In addition to safe care, CT is important for effective and efficient care. Effective care is individualized and accurate. It employs the correct interventions for the health situation at hand. Efficient care requires timely thinking so that resources are used appropriately. If Mr. Stone's nurses had been more effective in their thinking, they would have individualized their assessment, accurately diagnosed his risk for pneumonia right from the start, and implemented proper interventions. In addition, if Mr. Stone's nurses had used more CT, his hospital stay would have been shorter, thus saving time, money, and energy. In short, his care would have been more efficient. This scenario demonstrates the impact thinking has on patients and their significant others. CT makes a huge difference in patient care outcomes!

Why Is Thinking Important to Clinicians?

Clinicians make a jillion decisions every day. Most of those decisions are made in microseconds, but can have very serious consequences. Some decisions allow for more thinking time, consultation with others, and a search of other resources before coming to a conclusion. But all decisions must be accurate and made in a timely manner. Clinicians who employ all of the 17 CT dimensions automatically have more confidence in their reasoning. *Confidence* in reasoning allows nurses to speak their minds, to openly identify potential errors and "near misses," to contribute to team meetings, and to provide solid rationales for their decisions. Confidence empowers them to make valid contributions and decisions related to patient care and unit concerns. (See Box 4.3.)

Box 4.3

Why Is CT Important to Clinicians?

Thinking empowers decision-making skills.
Thinking enhances job satisfaction through professional integrity.
Thinking achieves expertise in practice.

CT is important to job satisfaction because it helps the clinician attain and maintain a professional nursing self-image. Even when parts of the nursing role are uncomfortable, good clinicians rely on professional ethics and *intellectual integrity* to reinforce their thinking. They derive job satisfaction from knowing that their thinking was actively engaged and the job was done to the best of their ability. One strategy to achieve such satisfaction is through *reflection* (Gustaffsson & Fagerberg, 2004).

The scenario in TACTICS 4.4 illustrates how CT empowers decision making and enhances job satisfaction.

TACTICS 4.4: Enhancing Decision-Making Skills and Job Satisfaction Through Professional Integrity

1. Read Scenario 4.2.
2. Which CT dimensions were used by Juan?
3. How do you think Juan felt about the situation?
4. How did Juan's CT affect both decision making and job satisfaction?

Scenario 4.2

Juan's Home Visit

Juan is a community health nurse. His home-care patient load today included 17-year-old Jenny and her 3-week-old newborn, Billy. This was Juan's first home visit with Jenny following up on a referral from the pediatrician's office because Billy had not gained weight since birth. Jenny was an unwed mother, living with her parents in a spacious, professionally decorated home in an upper middle class neighborhood. Jenny looked tired and interacted only minimally with Juan, and she rarely looked at the baby who was restless and fussy in his bassinet. Jenny's mother was home and she did most of the talking, explaining how she expected Jenny to take full responsibility for Billy's care. In fact, Jenny's parents both worked and were frequently out of town on business, but because of Juan's visit Jenny's mother stayed home today to assure the nurse that though the visit was well-intentioned, it was certainly not necessary.

Juan examined Billy and found some disturbing data. Billy had lost another 3 ounces and there were several dark areas on his back and legs. These markings had not been noted on the referral information.

Juan asked more questions. Jenny's mother assured him that Jenny was doing a fine job; they would be sure Billy got an extra feeding to gain his weight back; and all her children bruised easily so Billy probably inherited that trait.

Juan, however, had to make a tough decision. He didn't want to believe the baby was being abused; this was a "normal" looking family in a decent neighborhood. But he couldn't ignore the data: indications of ineffective maternal bonding, failure to thrive, and the apparent recent bruising all pointed to possible abuse. He also knew he was legally obligated to report suspected abuse. He was not comfortable with his decision to file a formal report, but he was confident it was the correct decision and he could justify his reasoning. Juan found out later that the nurse at the pediatrician's office had similar concerns, but she only had the original weight loss data to go on. She told Juan that she didn't want to bias his thinking, so she didn't share her suspicions with him until after his visit.

Discussion

The key thinking dimensions Juan used in this situation were *intellectual integrity* (although he did not want to believe the infant was being abused, he had to consider the evidence), *applying standards* (he was legally required to report suspected abuse), *confidence* (he trusted his reasoning ability), and *logical reasoning* (he believed he had adequate evidence to support his suspicions).

Juan very likely also felt shocked, uncomfortable, and annoyed. Shocked and uncomfortable that an upper-middle class family might be abusing a child; and annoyed that the nurse in the pediatrician's office had not been open about her suspicions before the visit. He probably believed he had been *open-minded* enough to collect accurate information even if he knew of the nurse's "hunch."

When Juan *reflected* on the situation, he could justify and support his decisions. He knew his judgment was sound. As an individual and a professional, he derived satisfaction from knowing he may have saved a life and provided an opportunity for a family to become more functional. He became a nurse because he wanted to help people and that goal was accomplished. By doing his job with compassion and *intellectual integrity* his behavior matched his role expectations, leading to job satisfaction.

Another way that CT benefits clinicians is by helping them move from novice to advanced beginner to competent to proficient and, ultimately, to expert (Benner, 1984). Throughout this process the clinician moves away from the context-free rules of novice decision making to more sophisticated levels of thinking. Thinking is essential to expert nurses, who can imagine the whole of a situation from a few details. They use reflection in action; they have learned to trust their intuitions. And they do all of this consistently. Expert nurses engage all 17 CT dimensions so naturally and with such ease that their decisions look effortless. The hard work of the thinking behind their actions is rarely apparent unless they have recognized how important it is to think out loud. Many experts don't recognize how fine-tuned thinking is, but they couldn't be experts without it. This level of thinking benefits patients as well as nurses.

Why Is CT Important to Educators?

Nurse educators derive all the benefits that clinicians do from CT and more. CT helps novice (and experienced) educators accept the reality that they do not need to know everything. This acceptance usually comes harder to the novice educator. Most experienced educators come to realize that their brains do not have enough RAM to store all needed information, and that the information they need to store keeps changing. With good CT habits of mind and skills educators can be comfortable saying "Let's go look that up" or

"That's a good question, but I'll have to get back to you with an answer" or "Gee, I don't know, but let's see if we can figure it out." Thinking helps educators accept that they don't know it all, but because of their CT, they have effective strategies to search for the best information. (See Box 4.4.)

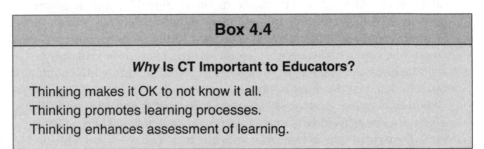

Box 4.4

Why Is CT Important to Educators?

Thinking makes it OK to not know it all.
Thinking promotes learning processes.
Thinking enhances assessment of learning.

CT helps both service-based and academic-based educators promote learning processes. Notice that we said learning, not teaching. Teaching can be simply imparting information to a passive recipient. Learning requires active engagement among the learner, the content, and the educator. CT helps the educator design such interactive learning processes, illuminating the connection between pieces of information and allowing learners to discover answers through their own use of CT. For example, instead of simply sharing the latest evidence-based guidelines on use of a new heparin-lock device with her staff, the staff development specialist provides the time and a place for focused dialogue, exploring the advantages and disadvantages of this new device. What are the challenges of using it? How is it best used in patient care? Does it meet guidelines? CT is important to create learning processes that maximize real behavior change and to transform information into useable *knowledge*.

CT also helps educators assess learning outcomes. For example, rather than selecting prepackaged assessment tools or educator-created competency check-offs for evaluation of learning, the critically thinking educator will examine existing tools to see how well they match with what needs to be learned. CT is needed to make those comparisons. For example, the Nursing Practice Laboratory Coordinator will anticipate how students should demonstrate competency in intramuscular injections. She will think about the answers to the following questions before she facilitates learning: What principles must the student articulate? What level of psychomotor skill must the student achieve? How can learning be designed to achieve the desired outcomes? What is the best way to assess that learning? These questions must be answered before the actual laboratory learning (and thinking) occurs with the students. This preteaching CT helps the coordinator design assessment tools that do the job they are intended to do. Without thinking about the assessment, as well as the learning, educators do only half of their thinking jobs. Thinking is the common denominator for service-based and academic-based educators if they want to promote learning that results in behavior change.

Why Is CT Important to IDT?

Effective interdisciplinary teams (IDTs): 1) are made up of members from more than one discipline or professional group, 2) are expected to pool their CT skills and habits of the mind to expand on ideas, and 3) consider all members as equal partners in thinking, including patients and significant others. Current evidence indicates that functional interdisciplinary teams are the ideal for achieving desired health outcomes (IOM, 2003) and experts have noted the need to improve team thinking as well as actions (Halpern, 1998; Sanderson, 2003).

Other teams—multidisciplinary teams, for example—also benefit from CT, of course. But because CT is so important to IDTs let us distinguish them from other healthcare teams: Multidisciplinary teams typically provide their discipline's perspective on patient situations, but do not necessarily engage in collective problem identification and decision making. IDTs do all of this, and more.

So, what is different about CT in IDTs and *why* is this thinking so important? We'll discuss the answers to these questions in Chapter 7, but to pique your interest, we have selected just three reasons why CT is so important to IDT. (See Box 4.5.)

Box 4.5

Why Is CT Important to the Interdisciplinary Team (IDT)?

Individual thinking provides the IDT with the raw material for problem identification and problem solving.

Team thinking provides the synergy to create ideas that individuals would not achieve independently.

Team thinking enhances group cohesion.

First, the thinking of the individual team members provides a wide range of raw material upon which team thinking can be built. Their CT, combined with their individual knowledge base and paradigms for problem identification and decision making, is an essential contribution to the team's overall functioning.

Second, the team can examine, discuss, and select options from a larger pool of information and "mix and match" options before making decisions. It is this pooling of ideas that leads to the synergistic thinking so valued in healthcare.

Third, team thinking is also important to group cohesion. Starting in the 1960s, the literature on group work and team work consistently identified group cohesion as essential to effective outcomes (Massello, 1998). Team thinking provides opportunities for developing trust and respect, both of which contribute to this group cohesion and, thus, to more effective outcomes—the goal of IDT work.

Summary of the First Ring of Stakeholders

Clinicians, educators, and IDTs compose the first ring of stakeholders orbiting our galaxy's center—patients and significant others. These stakeholders are in the first ring because their thinking has the most immediate impact on desired health outcomes for patients. Although educators do not always perform direct patient care, the students they supervise will, therefore, educators legitimately belong in this orbit. Not only does the CT of these stakeholders benefit patients and their significant others, it directly benefits the stakeholders themselves. Clinicians who use CT are empowered. Educators who use CT are comfortable not having all the answers. IDT members who use CT value and respect each other and their discipline's contributions to healthcare.

WHY IS CT IMPORTANT TO THE OTHER STAKEHOLDERS?

The thinking of stakeholders in the outer orbits affects patients and their significant others, clinicians, educators, and IDT members. We also emphasize the importance of CT to the stakeholders themselves because CT relates to their more immediate goals including unit functioning, survival of the organization, social policy, and professional responsibilities. Yet, these outer two rings of orbiting stakeholders also use CT to affect patient outcomes.

We have selected just a few reasons CT is important to each of them. As you read, see if you can think of additional reasons.

Why Is CT Important to Unit Managers?

Unit managers benefit from their own CT and the CT of others in many ways: better use of resources, achieving unit goals, and demonstrating quality of care on the unit. The thinking unit manager (and thinking staff) might use *creativity* to rethink how clean linen is delivered to the unit in order to save money, or *flexibility* to schedule IDT meetings at convenient times to develop goals and strategies. She might model *inquisitiveness* by working with staff to identify new safety policies and procedures to improve quality on the unit. She might use *reflection* to mentor peers and improve consistency in management approaches (Hyrkas, Koivula, Lehti, & Paunonen-Ilmonen, 2003). Managers' CT abilities have a huge impact on all stakeholders in our galaxy.

Why Is CT Important to Healthcare Administrators?

Administrators in charge of organizations such as hospitals, long-term care facilities, home care agencies, trauma centers, and outpatient clinics are primarily responsible for maintaining and developing their organizations and promoting quality service in a cost-effective way. CT is the only way to find solutions to what some view as polarized interests. For example, quality and cost-effectiveness are frequently viewed as opposites, yet CT can help reframe that perspective. Polarity management is one strategy for using CT to *analyze* commonalities and then find *creative* ways to deal with other issues (Yoder-Wise, 1995). *Transforming knowledge* is another CT essential for administrators whose organizations are moving toward more patient-centered care (Miller, Galloway, Coughlin, & Brennan, 2001). Hansten and Washburn (1999) noted administrators must have, "Advanced abilities to think critically . . . to improve clinical systems, decrease errors and sentinel events, and engage staff involvement to refine patient care systems" (p. 39).

Administration in healthcare is not confined to the practice setting. Administrators in institutions of higher education that teach health providers also need and benefit from CT. The setting may be different, but the needs are the same; CT is important in finding the balance between quality education and its cost. We don't have to tell you that healthcare education—particularly in medicine, nursing, pharmacy, and dentistry—is expensive. Remember the bumper sticker: "If you think education is expensive, try ignorance!" Maybe we should make a bumper sticker that says, "If you think thinking time is expensive, try healthcare without it!"

Why Is CT Important to Third-Party Payers?

Speaking of cost, this is where thinking is important to third-party payers—the insurance companies, Medicare, and Medicaid. Remember Mr. Stone, who developed pneumonia because of inadequate CT? Fortunately, his insurance covered the cost of his prolonged hospitalization, but that cost was unnecessary and a waste of resources. According to data collected by the Michigan Nurses' Association (MNA), "Hospital-acquired pneumonia among surgical patients may add between $22,390 and $28,505 per patient to hospital costs." (MNA, 2004).

Third-party payers must rely on CT to maintain their ability to pay for healthcare and keep their stockholders happy. They particularly depend on *analyzing* and *predicting* to do their jobs. They also recognize the importance of changing their thinking from a focus on short-term goals to what will occur over the long term. Pronovost (2004) described a plan currently being used by BlueCross and BlueShield in Michigan in which BC/BS worked with interdisciplinary teams from 107 ICUs to find ways to improve safety and save money. Other third-party payers will need to examine these problems more closely as the cost of healthcare, particularly of preventable conditions, rises.

Why Is CT Important to Healthcare Organizations, Governments, and the Healthcare Professions?

The outermost ring of our solar system of stakeholders contains the most complex organizations. CT at this level is very challenging and equally essential. Although at first glance these stakeholders may seem to have little impact on the day-to-day activities of healthcare organizations, in reality their CT is very important to clinicians and educators. The CT of healthcare organizations, governments, and the healthcare professions influences the policies, legislation, and standards that guide both practice and education. It has long-term effects on the day-to-day activities AND thinking of all stakeholders. Because these stakeholders have such a broad span of influence, they can use CT to see the "big picture" as well as the details, allowing them to design and implement policies that affect many people.

Healthcare organizations need to use CT consistently to function effectively and achieve their missions and goals, while maximizing their resources. For example, *creativity* helps them find better ways to organize staffing patterns. *Analysis* and *logical reasoning* help them examine infection patterns or track the rising costs of supplies. *Flexibility* helps them redirect services to meet changing customer needs.

All government organizations (both federal and state) that are mandated to protect the public welfare need at least *analysis, logical reasoning*, and *contextual perspective* to help accomplish their goals while balancing the demands of other activities, all competing for the same tax dollars. For example, *analysis* and *logical reasoning* can be used to determine why a state's mental health system is ranked lowest in the nation. *Contextual perspective* helps government groups understand how weather conditions affect the air conditioning needs of the growing numbers of citizens with chronic obstructive pulmonary disease.

Other healthcare professions also rely on all 17 CT dimensions to meet the criteria for their professional status. Those criteria will vary, depending on the source you use, but the basics of any profession include a code of ethics, a body of knowledge, higher education, and self-regulation (Haynes, Boese, & Butcher, 2004). How could one achieve a code of ethics without *reflection* and *logical reasoning*? How could one develop a body of knowledge without *analysis* and *inquisitiveness*? How could a professional organization design guidelines for a university curriculum without *perseverance* and *information seeking*? How could one manage self-regulation and accreditation standards without *applying standards*, *discriminating*, and *intellectual integrity*? *Contextual perspective* is essential as healthcare professions move toward interdisciplinary teamwork, learning from each other while maintaining their autonomous bodies of knowledge. You can probably cite examples for all the remaining CT dimensions.

WHAT MORE CAN BE DONE TO EMPHASIZE *WHY* CT IS IMPORTANT?

Something is only important if we value it. Words on paper do not create value. As Fullan (1993) said, "You can't mandate what matters" (p. 21). CT can never be mandated; the only successful activity is using mandates "as catalysts to reexamining" (p. 24) the current state of affairs, which can lead to value changes. This applies to the nursing and healthcare sectors very clearly. Clinicians who are expected to promote CT, but don't value it, may give lip service to its importance, but are not 1) going to commit the energy necessary for CT and 2) experience the role satisfaction that CT produces. Educators who expect to teach nursing and CT, but do not value thinking, will experience the same dilemmas.

So how can we help people learn to value CT? We start with Fullan's catalysts—words in mission statements, accreditation standards, and textbooks— and then we have to bring the words to life. And we do this by talking about CT every day, to nurture and cultivate ours and the CT of others. Consider the following scenario, in which a graduate student is explaining to his instructor how he modeled CT for a nursing student he was preceptoring on an inpatient medical surgical unit.

This scenario demonstrates *why talking* about your thinking makes it more real for your students (if you are an educator) or your staff (if you are a clinician). Because they cannot *see* your neurons firing, you have the responsibility to make CT overt. Once CT becomes overt through specific language, its value can be recognized.

Scenario 4.3

Modeling CT

A patient was admitted to an inpatient medical surgical unit for evaluation of cardiac arrhythmia. She had a history of mental illness as well. Recent symptoms included nausea, diarrhea, and a low-grade fever. This was the reflection the instructor shared with his graduate student:

> *I wanted the student to see how I was thinking through this problem and that it was OK to not have all the answers. The patient had a long history of bipolar disorder and had been taking lithium for several years successfully managing her disease. The staff told us she was also a bit of a hypochondriac and that this was the second time this month she was complaining of the flu. I told the student, "We have to be careful and not let our perceptions affect our data collection; we have to be **open-minded** from the beginning. Let's use some **inquisitiveness** here and find out from the patient what is happening. We need a little more **contextual perspective** so we need to get some historical information, a sense of what has been going on in her life recently, food allergies, and so on. I'm also wondering about the possibility of lithium toxicity. Go grab a drug book and let's check that out. What do you think? How do her lab values compare to the norms? Let's do some **analysis** here and look at all the pieces and then think about how they do or don't fit together. Think about it for a minute and tell me what dimensions of our thinking will be needed next?" We discovered that the patient was, in fact, having a toxic reaction to lithium. Her blood levels were over 1.5 mEq/L. She **wasn't** just being a hypochondriac. I really tried to use my CT words so that the student could see inside my brain. I had to figure this out all on my own—I want my student to have a head start.*

The challenge is to really talk about *thinking*, not just talk about *doing*! It takes practice, reflection, and peer feedback to get things rolling. The TACTICS activity below was designed to help clinicians and educators simulate, cultivate, and nurture their "talking about thinking."

TACTICS 4.5: Verbalizing CT so Others Will See the Value

Clinicians and Educators

This activity requires three people, paper and pencil, and maybe some colored highlighters. One person assumes the role of the educator; one person assumes the role of the staff member or student; and one person assumes the role of the observer. Ideally this activity could be video-taped, but it works equally well without taping. The activity can be re-peated by exchanging roles after the first time around.

Part I (5–10 minutes)

Educator: Your job is to select a teaching situation that will help your staff or students learn some aspect of nursing care but will also al-low you to model your thinking as you are modeling your explanation of care.

Staff/Student: Your job is to listen for the educator's CT messages and jot them down as you are learning.

Observer: Your job is to listen for both the educator's and the staff or student's thinking. Take notes that can be shared with the others later. Note: What words were used that reflect thinking? How many thinking words (*open-mindedness, confidence, analyzing, predicting,* etc.) were used in comparison to action words ("Next I need to flush the tubing")? Which of the educator's words represented thinking even if the vocabulary of the 17 CT dimensions was not used? Be as specific as possible as you take notes, you might want to keep a separate section of your notes where you can write down each of the verbalized CT dimensions.

Begin the exercise. After the 5–10 minutes, have each participant rate the Educator, using the following scale of 1–10 with 10 being the most.

How much of the teaching focused on doing? 1 2 3 4 5 6 7 8 9 10
How much of teaching focused on thinking? 1 2 3 4 5 6 7 8 9 10
How often were the 17 CT dimensions used? 1 2 3 4 5 6 7 8 9 10

What might the educator do differently the next time to more explicitly model thinking with CT words?

If you have highlighters, use them to mark the actual CT dimensions verbalized.

Part II (10–15 minutes)

Observer: Share your notes and your rankings with the others
Student/Staff: Share your notes and your rankings with the others
Educators: Share your notes and your rankings with the others

Discussion

How did everyone do? What did you discover about how your model-ing of thinking can be used the next time you teach CT?

Educators in any setting are expected to teach thinking. Teaching CT, however, requires one to accept that CT is a process, not simply more content. For example, when teaching the process of communication, we don't simply lecture on it, we model it, provide lots of opportunities to practice it, and have students overtly identify skills such as restatement, clarifying, and open-ended questions. We use process recordings to help students see those skill labels and patterns of use. Teaching CT must also be process-oriented. Reflection journals serve this purpose and are valuable tools to make thinking more overt.

Talking about thinking, as in the previous TACTICS exercise, helps us and others visualize thinking. Talking about thinking helps us recognize *why* CT is important to us and to our students, patients, organizations, and professions. Talking about CT, using CT terminology, can help us accomplish what organizational and professional mandates can only serve as catalysts for—valuing thinking.

PAUSE AND PONDER:
WHY DO YOU THINK CT IS IMPORTANT?

By now we hope you appreciate *why* CT is so important to the healthcare stakeholders, particularly *why* thinking is so important to clinicians and educators. CT is that important bridge we talked about in Chapter 2, transforming information to useful knowledge upon which patients and all the stakeholders can act. Without CT any attempts for safe, effective, efficient healthcare are meaningless.

Reflection Cues

- *Why* questions imply a search for reason, purpose, meaning, and value.
- *Why* and the thinking connected with *why* have triggered many important discoveries over the years.
- Many disciplines believe CT is important: medicine, engineering, law, business, education, aviation, and healthcare.
- Current matters requiring more or better CT include: the information explosion; dwindling resources; cost containment; third-party payer gatekeeping; morbidity and mortality data; patient safety and failure to rescue; and the emergent ethical dilemmas, such as right to life, prolongation of life without quality and stem cell research.
- Many stakeholders experience the consequences of thinking and not thinking: patients and significant others, clinicians, educators and interdisciplinary teams, unit managers, healthcare administrators, third-

party payers, healthcare organizations, governments, and healthcare professions.

- CT leads to safe, effective, and efficient care for patients.
- CT leads to empowered decision making, job satisfaction, and expertise in practice for clinicians.
- CT leads to realistic expectations and a focus on learning more than teaching.
- Clinicians and educators must begin to vocalize their CT to cultivate and nurture it in others.

References

Alverno College, Academics, Nursing (2004). Retrieved August 10, 2004, from http://www.alverno.edu/academics/nursing.html.

Benner, P. (1984). *From novice to expert: Power and excellence in nursing practice*. Menlo Park, CA: Addison-Wesley.

Brookfield, S. (1995). *Becoming a critically reflective teacher*. San Francisco: Jossey-Bass.

Brookfield, S. D. & Preskill, S. (1999). *Discussion as a way of teaching: Tools and techniques for democratic classrooms*. San Francisco: Jossey-Bass.

Critical Thinking Consortium (2004). Retrieved August 10, 2004, from http://www.critical thinking.org/.

Dreyfus, H. L. & Dreyfus, S. E. (1986). *Mind over machine: The power of human intuition and expertise in the era of the computer*. New York: The Free Press.

Famous Quotes, Einstein quotes. (n.d.). Retrieved August 8, 2004, from http://home.att.net/~quotations/einstein.html.

Fullan, M. (1993). *Change forces: Probing the depths of educational reform*. Bristol, PA: The Falmer Press.

Gustaffsson, C. & Fagerberg, I. (2004). Reflection, the way to professional development? *Journal of Clinical Nursing, 13*(3), 271–280.

Halpern, D. F. (1998). Teaching critical thinking for transfer across domains: Dispositions, skills, structure training, and metacognitive monitoring. *American Psychologist, 53*(4), 449–455.

Hansten, R. I. & Washburn, M. J. (1999). Individual and organizational accountability for developing critical thinking. *Journal of Nursing Administration, 29*(11), 39–45.

Haynes, L., Boese, T., & Butcher, H. (2004). *Nursing in contemporary society: Issues, trends, and transition to practice*. Upper Saddle River, NJ: Pearson Prentice Hall.

Hyrkas, K., Koivula, M., Lehti, K., & Paunonen-Ilmonen, M. (2003). Nurse managers' conceptions of quality management as promoted by peer supervision. *Journal of Nursing Management, 11*, 48–58.

Institutes, Centers and Societies, Nursing (2004). Retrieved August 10, 2004, from http://www.austhink.org/critical/pages/nursing.html.

Institute of Medicine (IOM). (2003). *Health professions education: A bridge to quality*. Washington, DC: The National Academies Press.

Institute of Medicine (IOM). (2004). *Keeping patients safe: Transforming the work environment for nurses.* Washington, DC: The National Academies Press.

Marzano, R. & Pickering, D. (1997). *Dimensions of learning teacher's manual.* (2nd ed.). Alexandria, VA: Association for Supervision and Curriculum Development.

Massello, D. J. (1998). Operations management: Administering the program. In K. J. Kelly-Thomas (Ed.), *Clinical and Nursing Staff Development: Current Competent, Future Focus,* 2nd ed. (pp. 337–364). Philadelphia: Lippincott.

Michigan Nurses' Association. (2004). *The business case for reducing patient-to-nurse staff ratios and eliminating mandatory overtime for nurses.* Lansing, MI: Public Policy Associates, Inc.

Miller, J., Galloway, M., Coughlin, C., & Brennan, E. (2001). Care-centered organizations, Part I: Governance. *Journal of Nursing Administration, 31*(2), 67–73.

National League for Nursing Accrediting Commission. (2003). *Accreditation manual for postsecondary and higher degree programs in nursing: Interpretive guidelines by program type.* New York: Author.

Paul, R. (1992). *Critical thinking: What every person needs to survive in a rapidly changing world.* Santa Rosa, CA: Foundation for Critical Thinking.

Pronovost, P. J. (2004, March). *Healthcare safety and quality revolution.* Paper presented at the American Association of Colleges of Nursing Spring Annual Meeting, Fairmont Hotel, Washington, DC.

Sanderson, H. (2003). Implementing person-centered planning by developing person-centered teams. *Journal of Integrated Care, 11*(3), 18–25.

Scheffer, B. K. (2001). Nurse educators' perspectives on their critical thinking: Snapshots from their personal and professional lives. (Doctoral dissertation, *Dissertation Abstracts International, 2001). 62,* 2B, 786.

Schon, D. A. (1983). *The reflective practitioner: How professionals think in action.* New York: Basic Books.

Senge, P. M. (1990). *The fifth discipline: The art & practice of the learning organization.* New York: Doubleday.

Wiggins, G. & McTighe, J. (2001). *Understanding by design.* Upper Saddle River, NJ: Merrill Prentice Hall.

Yoder-Wise, P. S. (1995). *Leading and managing in nursing.* St. Louis: Mosby.

CHAPTER 5

The *How*, *When*, and *Where* of Critical Thinking for Clinicians and Educators

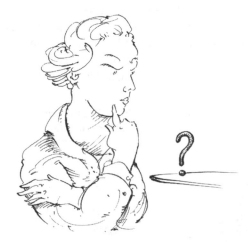

You can probably tell that our scheme of the *what, who, why,* and so on looks good to start with but gets very muddy as we move along. We gave up trying to keep them separated and have combined the last three of the six—*how, when,* and *where*—together. It was difficult to keep the *who* separated from *what* and *why*, but it is virtually impossible to discuss these last three out of the context of critical thinking (CT). If nothing else, CT is contextual in nature. No matter what it is that crosses our mind, it does so because something (*what*), somewhere (*where*), and at some time (*when*), triggered that thought. *How* one thinks about anything, therefore, is influenced by the context (*when* and *where*) of that thought. That thinking, in turn, affects what happens relative to that issue or problem. The process is dynamic and reflexive.

CURRENT CHALLENGES AND SOLUTIONS FOR HEALTHCARE DELIVERY

No*where* is the *how* of CT more needed than in the healthcare arena, and the *when* is definitely now. Healthcare is faced with many challenges these days. In its 2001 report, *Crossing the Quality Chasm: A New Health System for the 21st Century,* the U.S. Institute of Medicine (IOM) called healthcare professionals to action to improve patient care quality and safety. One recommendation was to convene an interdisciplinary summit to recommend approaches to accomplish these improvements. That summit, which met in 2002, culminated in *Health Professions Education: A Bridge to Quality* (IOM, 2003). It found that one major way we can affect practice is to change how we prepare healthcare practitioners. We need to lay better groundwork.

"All health professionals should be educated to deliver patient-centered care as members of an interdisciplinary team, emphasizing evidence-based practice, quality improvement approaches and informatics" (IOM, 2003, p. 3). The relationship among those five areas is shown in Figure 5.1.

Figure 5.1   Working in Interdisciplinary Teams, Using Evidence-Based Practice and Informatics for Patient-Centered Care and Quality Improvement

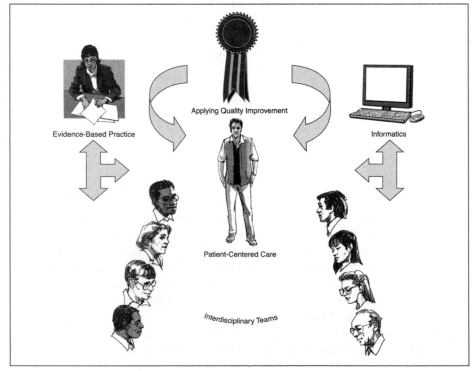

Box 5.1

Core Competencies for a New Vision for Health Professions Education
(IOM, 2003, p. 4)

1. **Provide patient-centered care**—identify, respect, and care about patients' differences, values, preferences, and expressed needs; relieve pain and suffering; coordinate continuous care; listen to, clearly inform, communicate with, and educate patients; share decision making and management; and continuously advocate disease prevention, wellness, and promotion of healthy lifestyles, including a focus on population health.
2. **Work in interdisciplinary teams**—cooperate, collaborate, communicate, and integrate care in teams to ensure that care is continuous and reliable.
3. **Employ evidence-based practice**—integrate best research with clinical expertise and patient values for optimum care, and participate in learning and research activities to the extent feasible.
4. **Apply quality improvement**—identify errors and hazards in care; understand and implement basic safety design principles, such as standardization and simplification; continually understand and measure quality of care in terms of structure, process, and outcomes in relation to patient and community needs; and design and test interventions to change processes and systems of care, with the objective of improving quality.
5. **Utilize informatics**—communicate, manage knowledge, mitigate error, and support decision making using information technology.

To live up to that vision, a set of five core competencies was advocated for all health professions. *Competency* was defined as "the habitual and judicious use of communication, knowledge, technical skills, clinical reasoning, emotions, values and reflection in daily practice" (Hundert, as cited in IOM, 2003, pp. 3–4). Box 5.1 includes the definitions of the five competencies. As you can see, specific actions outlined in each definition fall into the communication, technical skills, clinical reasoning, emotions, values, and reflection categories of competence.

What Are Competencies?

We want to make sure that everyone understands what constitutes competencies or competency-based performance, because there are many misconceptions about these terms. By using the word "competencies," the IOM was focusing on summative behaviors that they want, even expect, to see in practice. Competencies are very specific end-points that can be assessed; they are more than just a general list of areas for improvement. The use of competency language in the IOM's recommendations makes a stronger statement, beyond a mere focus shift in healthcare delivery and education. They expect providers to be consistently competent in their performance in these five areas. Note the phrase "habitual and judicious use" in the quote on page 77.

Bargagliotti, Luttrell, and Lenburg (1999), citing Lenburg's earlier work, provided this definition: "Competency-based performance evaluation is defined as a criterion-referenced, summative evaluation process that assesses a participant's actual ability to meet a predetermined set of performance standards under controlled conditions and protocols" (section 1, para. 4). They noted the difference between this type of evaluation and traditional check-off methods in which a set of steps is demonstrated. Competency-based evaluations focus on evidence of effective implementation of specified skills; critical elements are demonstrated, but not necessarily in a step-by-step format. It's a bottom-line, real-world view, not a set of textbook steps. In short, it's all about performance.

CRITICAL THINKING AND COMPETENCIES

While the actual term *critical thinking* is never used in the IOM competencies, words that are close cousins certainly appear in these performance ideals. The definition of competency cited above speaks directly to *clinical reasoning, knowledge, values,* and *reflection.* Looking at all competencies, we see words like *sharing decision making* for patient-centered care; *integrating best research* when employing evidence-based practice; *understanding* quality and *designing* interventions in applying quality improvement; *managing knowledge* and supporting *decision making* with informatics (IOM, 2003). In short, CT seems to be a necessary prerequisite to meeting the core competencies and is threaded throughout each of the five. We will link specific dimensions of CT to these five core competencies as we explore the thinking needed to make them a reality.

A PICTURE OF CHANGES IN HEALTHCARE DELIVERY AND EDUCATION

Clearly evident in the IOM's vision is a move away from status quo behavior in healthcare education and practice and toward a focus on context-bound thinking (the how, when, and where). The quality of clinical practice will improve and there will be more collaboration among providers and with patients. Decisions will be based on evidence found through current informatics rather than on tradition. In the IOM view, these practice changes will occur through changes in health professions' education practices. We will begin our discussion of the *how* and *where*, then, with changes in educational systems.

There are many driving forces for change in practice arenas, such as cost containment, consumer demands, and new information. However, without a concomitant change in health professions education, that change will take longer (an important *when* consideration) and be less embedded in the values of clinicians. Also, because of the immediate demands of the practice arena, service-based educators will very likely feel the pressures to change more quickly than academic-based educators.

Changes in Teaching and Learning Within a Thinking Framework

Let's consider how teaching and learning are approached in service settings as compared to academic settings because, while teaching/learning principles and approaches are used in both, the nature of the settings (*where*) makes a difference sometimes to the related issues. Box 5.2 compares some of those key differences.

Service-based educators often have to fit their teaching of required, updated information into short, variable time slots to accommodate various shifts of nurses. Academic-based educators generally have structured class or clinical time that lasts anywhere from one to eight hours. Time and schedules certainly make a difference in the techniques used to teach clinicians versus nursing students.

Box 5.2

Differences Between Academic- and Service-Based Education

Factor	Academic-Based	Service-Based
Time blocks for teaching	Structured	Variable
Amount of time in blocks	Hours	Minutes
Mix of novice to expert	More homogeneous	More heterogeneous
Mix of students	Nursing students	Nursing and unlicensed personnel
Focus on knowledge	Knowledge more than practice	Practice more than knowledge
Context	More noncontextual	More contextual
Teaching environment	Mostly classrooms	Variable spaces

Service-based educators often deal with very heterogeneous groups—experienced nurses, novice nurses, and unlicensed assistive personnel (UAP). This creates additional challenges, as the language used in teaching and the expectations of the group must be modified and leveling information must play a part. In spite of these differences, both practice- and academic-based educators do use some similar teaching/learning approaches, and thus change in educational offerings, as well as delivery, will occur in both settings. Service-based educators, with their less-structured teaching situations, may find these changes easier to deal with. Educators in academic settings may experience more challenges due to traditions.

How these changes in education occur is where CT comes in: we must change our thinking. To meet the five core competencies, education cannot be carried out in the tradition of educators handing down information to learners. Instead, academic faculty and service-based educators will need to help students become active knowledge seekers rather than passive information receivers (Fig. 5.2). This type of teaching and learning is a collaborative effort, not the one-up, one-down configuration of the traditional authoritarian teaching.

How change in teaching/learning will occur will not be easy. Frederic Moore Binder, former President of Hartwick College (Gaie's excellent alma mater) recently cited this old adage: "Changing a college curriculum is like trying to

---

Figure 5.2   Nurses as Knowledge Seekers

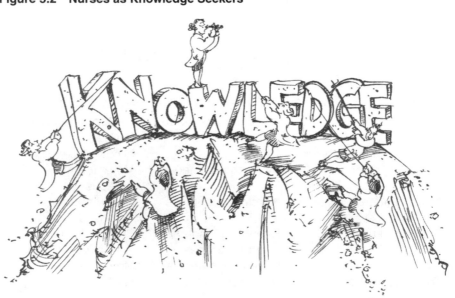

move a cemetery" (2000, para. 5). Perhaps service-based educators have less "buried" patterns, but we'll bet you can relate. As educators who have struggled through curriculum changes, we can attest to the truth of that cemetery analogy.

We have a long tradition of teachers being authorities and all-knowing. Students come through an education system that largely uses this hierarchical model of teaching; they expect to be takers of information. How, then, can nurse leaders and educators promote knowledge-seeking behaviors? We are talking about a teaching/learning paradigm shift. That sounds like a big deal, and we'll discuss that shortly, but first let's focus on some easily overlooked but vital "small" things.

Make Some Small Changes

Some students are affected by seemingly simple comments or actions. Look at Box 5.3 for a list of such simple comments and nonverbal behaviors that can either promote or squelch CT.

TACTICS 5.1: Promoting CT or Knowledge-Seeking Behavior

Clinicians

Using Box 5.3, reflect on your interactions with other staff over the past two days. How often have you made comments from the left column of the box and how often from the right? Be honest now!! Think about how you feel when you hear comments from each side of that box.

Educators

Using Box 5.3, think about your teaching situation in the past two months. How often have you made comments from the left column of the box and how often from the right? Be honest now! Alternatively, ask students to list what they think are the most and least productive teacher comments promoting knowledge-seeking behaviors. Use the responses as a self-inventory of the comments you make when teaching.

Discussion

You probably remember some of the CT-promoting and CT-squelching comments directed at you during your education. They stick in your mind, don't they? Especially the squelching ones. It's frightening to acknowledge the potential impact of our small comments, but it's healthy to contemplate how our behavior might help or hinder knowledge-seeking behavior.

Box 5.3

CT-Promoting and -Squelching Comments and Behaviors

CT-Promoting Comments and Behaviors	CT-Squelching Comments and Behaviors
• That's an interesting question.	• What a dumb question!
• There's no such thing as a dumb question.	• Don't you know that?
• Do you have a different idea how to do this?	• You should know that!
• Let's explore this.	• We've always done it this way.
• Let's think this through.	• That's the wrong way to do that.
• I'm not sure; can we figure this out?	• That'll never work here.
• Don't believe everything you read or hear.	• Just do it this way.
• Show me how you came to that conclusion.	• Why do you have to make everything so complicated?
• Can we look at this from a different angle?	• That will never fit in our budget.
• What do you think?	• Just memorize it.
• Walk me through your thinking on this.	• Stop with the questions, already!
• Tell me about what you learned here.	• Because I said so, that's why!
• Let's see what others have to say.	• If you're so sure of yourself, you figure it out.
• That's one option; let's see what other ways might also work.	• Mistakes are not tolerated here.
• What are some possible outcomes of that approach?	• Let's get moving; we don't have all day.
• That was a great example of how you used _____ (insert the CT dimension used, such as *inquisitiveness*).	• I can't believe you don't know that by now.
• That's a good idea; let's expand on it to make it even better.	• Come on, use your brain here!
• Use a neutral voice tone.	• It's too complicated to explain.
• Use an enthusiastic voice tone.	• I can't believe you said/did that!
• Sit silently and patiently.	• Roll eyes
	• Smirk
	• Big sighs
	• Scowl
	• Foot-tapping or finger-tapping
	• Other nonverbal demonstrations of anger, frustration, irritation
	• Look at one's watch frequently

Bigger Changes

Now, let's examine the bigger guns of teaching/learning approaches that will transform health professions' education in the 21st century. The philosopher John Dewey wrote *Democracy and Education* in 1916. Because his wisdom stands the test of time, and because he links thinking and action, Dewey's ideas have particular relevance for teaching and learning in health-care. Consider this gem from Dewey that will make you sit up and take note: "Information severed from thoughtful action is dead, a mind-crushing load" (1966, p. 153). Think about that quote the next time you write exam items. Do you want a simple recall of information or a more cognitively sophisticated application item? For those of you who hunger for more of Dewey's thoughts on education and thinking, we've compiled some "Dewey Diamonds" in Box 5.4.

Dewey's ideas underpin the problem-based learning (PBL) movement made popular by McMaster University in Ontario, Canada, and in common use worldwide today (Rideout, 2001). This student-centered approach to learning

---

Box 5.4

Dewey Diamonds
(The first bold lines are our translations. Sorry, Dewey.)

The quotes are from Dewey, J. (1966). Democracy and Education. New York: The Free Press (Original work published 1916, Macmillan Company)

Don't be too academic.
"Hence the first approach to any subject in school, if thought is to be aroused and not words acquired, should be as unscholastic as possible." (p. 154)

Both thinking without action and action without thinking get you nowhere.
"Thinking which is not connected with increase of efficiency in action, and with learning more about ourselves and the world in which we live, has something the matter with it just as thought. And skill obtained apart from thinking is not connected with any sense of the purposes for which it is to be used. It consequently leaves a man at the mercy of his routine habits and of the authoritative control of others." (p. 152)

Some people think you can improve thinking separately from what you do.
"[T]hinking is often regarded both in philosophic theory and in educational practice as something cut off from experience, and capable of being cultivated in isolation." (p. 153)

(continues)

Box 5.4 *(continued)*

Teachers, don't make things too hard or too simple.
"A large part of the art of instruction lies in making the difficulty of new problems large enough to challenge thought, and small enough so that, in addition to the confusion naturally attending the novel elements, there shall be luminous familiar spots from which helpful suggestions may spring." (p. 157)
Education is all about thinking.
"[T]he important thing is that thinking is the method of an educative experience. The essentials of method are therefore identical with the essentials of reflection." (p. 163)
Lectures on topics out of context are boring.
"[U]nder the influence of the conception of the separation of mind and material, method tends to be reduced to a cut and dried routine, to following mechanically prescribed steps." (p. 169)
Some teachers think you're a troublemaker if you ask questions.
"Exorbitant desire for uniformity of procedure and for prompt external results are the chief foes which the open-minded attitude meets in school. The teacher who does not permit and encourage diversity of operation in dealing with questions is imposing intellectual blinders upon pupils—restricting their vision to the one path the teacher's mind happens to approve." (p. 175)
It's not all about quick answers.
"The zeal for 'answers' is the explanation of much of the zeal for rigid and mechanical methods." (p. 175)
Some people still want someone to just give them the answers.
"Men still want the crutch of dogma, of beliefs fixed by authority, to relieve them of the trouble of thinking and the responsibility of directing their activity by thought." (p. 339)

---

links learning to action in that students are directed by relevant problems or issues rather than a set of topics defined by the teacher. Independent inquiry and reflection are important thinking components of this approach. (Remember, we started this book with a FAQ chapter because we believe questions are the best place to start a thinking journey.)

There are also many references to Dewey in Wiggins and McTighe's *Understanding by Design* (1998). They differentiated real understanding (that which uses learning in new ways) from knowledge that is "superficial, rote, out-of-context and easily tested" (p. 40). We want to promote real understanding, which Wiggins and McTighe viewed as having six facets: "When we truly understand, we can . . . explain . . . interpret . . . apply . . . have perspective . . .

can empathize . . . [and] have self-knowledge" (p. 44). Have you ever said, the best way to learn something is to teach it? Look at those six facets and think about the last time you spent a lot of time and energy preparing a lesson. You probably drew upon each of those six facets. A little later in this chapter we're going to discuss the benefits of picturing yourself teaching something as a way of learning. We'll revisit the six facets then.

Another recent take on Dewey's ideals is Barr and Tagg's article (1995), which clearly identifies the differences between teaching and learning. For example, teaching implies a hierarchy; learning is done in collaboration. Teaching implies covering material; learning implies performance outcomes. Teaching implies that "knowledge exists out there"; learning implies that "knowledge exists in each person's mind and is shaped by individual experience." Teaching implies that "knowledge comes in chunks and bits delivered by instructors"; learning implies that "knowledge is constructed, created, 'gotten' " (p. 43).

In today's healthcare world, where things change almost by the minute, we need to aim for the kind of understanding that allows for transfer of information to fit new situations—what we call *transforming knowledge*. This is what Perry (1970) called "relativism," where knowledge is contextual and relative and multiple perspectives fit into a big picture. This relativism is in contrast to "dualism," where there are right and wrong answers and the world is seen in absolute categories. In nursing we are most familiar with these ways of viewing situations and gaining knowledge from Benner's work (1984). Benner defined these differences as existing between novices and expert nurses. From her work, we have learned to do all we can to move nurses away from novice dualism to the contextual thinking of experts.

Old dualistic teaching and learning methods just don't cut it. Clinicians cannot learn about new medications and procedures and expect that information to remain static; it will change, for example, as research reveals better procedures or as medications are shown to be valuable for off-label uses. Clinicians must be able to converse intelligently about new information with the healthcare team and with patients and families.

Educators shouldn't just test students for their recall of textbook information. Who cares what you know today if you won't be able to use that knowledge tomorrow when the context changes? We must help students process information and use it to define their own knowledge. We must move away from shoveling content at students and move toward learning partnerships focused on students discovering things for themselves. And we must develop new habits of the mind to help students do the same. "The development of understanding greatly depends on such attitudes and habits of mind as open-mindedness, self-discipline (autonomy), tolerance for ambiguity, and reflectiveness" (Wiggins & McTighe, 1998, p. 171).

In the academic side of nursing, any suggestion related to changing how content is taught generally sends seasoned faculty running, holding their lecture notes close to their hearts. We are too focused on teaching specific content, fearing that students will not learn content unless it is taught directly. Debates over content often get dichotomized because of the assumption that content and process are parallel and mutually exclusive. This leads to the idea that one must teach either process *or* content. For those teaching undergraduate students, one of the driving forces behind a rigid focus on content is that students must pass the NCLEX. This kind of thinking presupposes that students will not learn content if it is not spoon-fed to them. Does that make any sense? No. We are caught in the providing-information paradigm.

So what needs to be done? Starting with simple steps first, we need to redefine the process of acquiring knowledge and understanding (content). A teaching method is not the same as a learning process. Certainly, some teaching methods do seem to promote learning better than others and we'll discuss some of those shortly. But learning is a whole other process and it doesn't matter much what we teach and how we do it, if no one learns.

We should also clarify what we mean by "content" and "process": Content is information and process is what we do with that information. There's certainly a necessary marriage of the two in a practice discipline. However, that's too facile; we need to expand on the idea of content or knowledge. We need to distinguish between the acquisition of information and the process of true learning. True learning means internalizing information and transforming it into knowledge until it becomes part of the learner's ideas. Only then can the learner use that knowledge meaningfully (such as for patient-care situations). In this context, Dewey's observations are helpful. He said that we don't convey ideas. Ideas form as we do something in our heads with the facts told to us. When facts are shared,

> the communication may stimulate that other person to realize the question for himself and to think out a like idea, or it may smother his intellectual interest and suppress his dawning effort at thought. But what he directly gets cannot be an idea. Only by wrestling with the conditions of the problem at first hand, seeking and finding his own way out, does he think (1966, pp. 159–160).

If that doesn't stimulate you to plan interactive teaching, nothing will! We'll bet clinicians are nodding in agreement at this point, though educators may still be a bit skeptical. That's because clinicians are focused on using knowledge, not teaching it. Anyone who uses knowledge knows it's necessary to have it in idea form—what Wiggins and McTighe (1998) called real understanding—that can be used in a variety of ways. Ask clinicians how they learn best and most will say by practicing or using something. In other words, they are thinking of ideas, not facts. They have done something with what they learned. They have internalized the information so they can use it. Educators need to take a lesson from clinicians and focus on what their students will be doing with the information they are receiving; then educators can adapt their teaching methods to the realities of healthcare practice.

TECHNIQUES TO PROMOTE THINKING AND KNOWLEDGE PROCESSING

How about some discussion of teaching techniques to promote thinking and the processing of knowledge? Thankfully, there are many teaching method resources out there for educators these days. Our favorite is what we call the "CAT" book (*Classroom Assessment Techniques*) by Angelo and Cross (1993). Even though it says "classroom," we think service educators will find it useful, too. Another helpful guide is by Billings and Halstead (2005). We have listed some of the techniques adapted from those sources in Box 5.5. Note that these are all interactive approaches.

Box 5.5

Teaching Techniques to Promote Processing and Internalization of Knowledge

(*Adapted from Angelo & Cross, 1993; ~Adapted from Billings & Halstead, 2005)

__Muddiest Point__: After presenting content, have students write on cards the muddiest point and hand them in anonymously; the teacher then discusses each of those points.

__One-Sentence Summary__: Have students sum up what they just learned in one sentence. Then, in groups, have them explain why they came up with that sentence.

__One-Word Summary__: A variation on the one-sentence summary, students choose one word and explain why that word summarizes the idea.

__Concept or Mind Maps__: Students map out ideas and the connections among them, questions, answers, and so on, in some way that is meaningful to them.

__Student-generated test questions__: Students come up with test questions. These can be collected and used for tests/quizzes.

__Minute Paper__: At the end of teaching session, students are asked to answer a question, such as: "What was the most important thing you learned today?" or "What are you most curious to learn more about?" Students are given a minute to write an answer.

(continues)

Box 5.5 *(continued)*

Empty Outline or Empty Mind Map: The teacher gives students a partially completed outline or map; they need to fill in the blanks.

Memory Matrix: Students set up a grid with some ideas across the top and some down the side; they then fill in the squares to show relationships.

~**Algorithms:** Break tasks into yes/no steps to solve complex problems.

~**Argumentation/Debate:** Promotes logical reasoning and open-mindedness as students debate controversial issues. Works well when students have to argue the side opposite from their view.

~**Case Studies/Scenarios:** Use to teach content; have students share cases with similar or different parts.

~**Collaborative Learning:** Work groups for assignments or problem solving.

~**Newspaper Analysis:** Students analyze something written for the lay public; determine/critique sources of information; discuss relevance to nursing.

~**Reflection Projects/Logs:** Have students reflect on something, focusing specifically on their thinking.

Many of these teaching techniques discussed can also be used to assess CT competencies. If we view CT as just one of many competencies, then we need to be teaching so that students will be able to demonstrate their CT. Chapter 12 is all about assessing CT, so we'll limit our discussion here to making sure that you link assessment with teaching and learning. Box 12.2 will give you more ideas for teaching methods, although in that chapter we call them methods of assessing CT. So, for now, consider Chapter 12 an annex to Chapter 5.

Teaching as Learning

One of our favorite questions to undergraduate nursing students is this: "How would you explain that to a patient?" Think about that. Inevitably, nurses have to impart most of their knowledge to patients. Remember our discussion of Wiggins and McTighe's (1998) six facets of true understanding—explain, interpret, apply, have perspective, empathize, have self-knowledge. If those ring true in your mind you will agree that one of the best ways to learn something is to teach it to someone else. And having to teach someone who does not have your working vocabulary will make that an even more valuable learning experience, because now you have to translate the message, too. To do that, you *really* need to know it.

For our clinician readers, how often do you teach things to patients? Most of you will answer "continuously." Each day, as you learn new things, think about how you would effectively explain these things to a patient. Paolo Freire, the educational philosopher we quoted in Chapter 1, said this beautifully: "Whoever teaches learns in the act of teaching, and whoever learns teaches in the act of learning" (1998, p. 31).

Learning in the Workplace

In Chapter 11 we will discuss the realities of practice today and tomorrow, but here we'd like to sow the seeds for the learning environment. Carole Estabrooks (2003), in her discussion of using research in practice, character-ized nurses as generating knowledge within their "communities of practice" (p. 60). People don't learn in isolation; they do it with others. Nurses produce knowledge, as well as use it, in their workplaces every day. We don't think Dewey would be surprised to read this, especially if he considered the huge amount of knowledge that nurses must learn and use daily.

This idea of integrating learning and the practicalities of practice is echoed in Carkhuff's (1996) advocacy of reflective learning through the use of work/learning groups in the workplace. This approach is very helpful for service-based educators who want to move from the old goals of adaptive learning that focus on survival and maintenance, to a generative learning model, based on creativity and continuous learning (Watkins & Marsick, 1993). Carkhuff provided an excellent example of reflective group learning: While checking the competency of nurses to correctly identify and locate equipment on a crash cart, several nurses were unable to meet the criteria. Rather than re-teach the crash cart criteria, the staff educator encouraged the group to reflect upon and discuss why it was difficult to do this job without error. Together they came up with strategies to increase their competency. The keys to the success of this approach are that the learning was problem-based, learner directed, contextual, and reflective.

Reflection in Practice

We'd like to talk more about the value of reflection, not just as a teaching/learning tool, but also as a way to increase clinicians' CT. A word to clinicians: in the last few pages we've focused on educators, but it would be useful here for you to consider the thinking challenges you deal with daily. You probably do not practice as you once did because of the rapid pace of change in the healthcare arena. "Reflection in practice" is how Schon (1983) referred to this, a wonderful idea, which is poignantly relevant today. Schon advocated that practitioners think about what they are doing and thinking while in the midst of action—to be "reflective practitioners" in response to changes in their professions. Although healthcare professionals were one of his intended audiences, he cited many professionals who have experienced a "crisis of confidence" because of "the mismatch of traditional patterns of practice and knowledge [and the] . . . complexity, uncertainty, instability, uniqueness, and value conflict" of the practice arena (p. 18).

This complexity and uncertainty are especially found in what Schon called the "swampy lowland where situations are confusing 'messes' incapable of technical solution" (p. 42). Whoa! Does that sound like a typical *when* and *where* for nurses or what, eh? Schon also said that those who choose the swampy lowland "deliberately involve themselves in messy but crucially important problems and, when asked to describe their methods of inquiry, they speak of experience, trial and error, intuition, and muddling through" (p. 43). Can something be done to help clinicians "muddle through" better? Schon's answer is reflection.

How can clinicians use reflection to meet the goals that the IOM has advocated for practice? First and foremost you must focus on thinking—not as a phenomenon separate from daily work, but as it is joined with action. Now, don't get the idea here that nurses can ever practice without thinking. That is a scary thought. However, reflection in action is thinking about the thinking *and* the action as one is actively working. That reflection is necessary because of the changing nature of healthcare. What worked yesterday won't necessarily work today; what we did yesterday is not necessarily what we should be doing today. Thinking and acting are linked out of necessity; we don't have the luxury of sitting back and doing our thinking after the fact, nor would we be comfortable doing that. However, because it is so easy to concentrate on action rather than on the thinking, we need reminders to think.

How Does Reflection in Action Work?

At the risk of being prescriptive, we've come up with a list of questions that clinicians should ask themselves as they reflect. (See Box 5.6.) As you see, they are essentially based on the CT habits of the mind and skills that we have already discussed. Now, would each clinician reflect on these things in a linear, check-list kind of way? Of course not. But, it's helpful to have such a list to help us think about things fully.

TACTICS 5.2: Reflection in Action

Clinicians

Think about your most recent clinical day. Now think of a specific patient encounter or team meeting. Using the questions in Box 5.6, reflect

---

Box 5.6

Suggestions for Clinicians' Reflection in Action

Am I . . .

reasonably sure of my thinking here?

taking into account the total context of this situation?

considering more creative, better approaches?

being too rigid? Too loose?

asking all the questions I should be asking?

using any preconceived notions that might be wrong?

going with my gut reactions or ignoring them?

closing my mind off to any possibilities?

sticking with this long enough or is it time to just make a decision and get on with it?

breaking this down enough so I'm seeing all the pieces and how they fit together?

forgetting any important rules here?

seeing the patterns and details?

missing anything?

making conclusions based on solid data?

able to predict where this is going?

adapting my knowledge to this situation?

---

on these events. Pay attention to how comfortable you are with reflection. Try to picture yourself in the midst of what was happening. Were you reflective at the time? As you recall the situation, do things occur to you now that you didn't consider while the event was happening?

Discussion

If the checklist idea seems a bit scripted to you, think about other ways to promote reflective practice. Perhaps this real-life situation will spark your creativity.

We asked our nurse practitioner colleague, Jane Duerr, to describe her reflection in action. She talked about *where, when,* and *how* to reflect. (OK, so we prompted her with those words . . . nevertheless, this is what she said.)

I try to reflect with another clinician if I can because I think better when I can bounce ideas off someone else. I do that in several ways— both structured and informally. On the structured side, the nurse prac- titioners at my office get together for breakfast on a regular schedule to talk about practice issues. We make a point of not turning that into a complaining session about things we dislike, but, rather, we focus on things we've seen in practice that we're concerned with, new information we've found and so forth—real collaborative communication. The physicians and nurse practitioners also have a journal club where we reflect on our practice relative to the latest research findings. Less structured reflection occurs in the corridors and lunchroom; sometimes I call one of the docs or nurses to bounce ideas off them in the middle of the day.

I also reflect with families and patients. Sometimes sitting down and going over things with them allows me to think aloud; we can think together and often come up with better actions than I would have come up with alone. It's very easy to forget that patients and families are there, too.

As to where I reflect, it's everywhere, especially places where I can find some solitude. I go into the lab, find an empty office, I do a lot of reflection in my car on the way home or to and from settings. I often take a longer route home so I can have more thinking time.

The challenge to you who are clinicians is this: How are you managing reflection in practice? Do you do it enough? Where do you do it? Do you need to reflect on your reflection?

 PAUSE AND PONDER: THINK AHEAD TO CHANGE

In this chapter, we've discussed how educators and clinicians need to grow to make sure that the competencies of providing patient-centered care, working in interdisciplinary teams, employing evidence-based practice, applying quality improvement, and using informatics become the norm of health care.

This chapter is a bookend on one side of the next five chapters that address the IOM competencies. In Chapter 11, the other bookend, we will revisit some of the ideas introduced here when we consider the day-to-day realities of healthcare practice and education. In this chapter we described many overt and covert messages about the necessity for change. We'll pick up that theme in Chapter 11, expanding on what thinking is necessary to survive the inevitable complexities of change in healthcare delivery and education.

Reflection Cues

- The *how*, *when*, and *where* of CT for clinicians and educators are intrinsically interconnected: the *where* is healthcare practice and education; the *when* is today and tomorrow. What remains is to figure out the best *how*.

- The Institute of Medicine has issued a challenge for health professions to deliver patient-centered care as members of an interdisciplinary team—emphasizing evidence-based practice, quality improvement approaches, and informatics—and for healthcare educators to produce clinicians who can achieve this task (IOM, 2003, p. 3).

- Meeting the IOM's challenge will require major changes in the practice and education of health professionals.

- Education must move away from the status quo of traditional teaching and start focusing on active learning rather than rote memorization.

- Students must become finders of knowledge, not takers of information.

- Knowledge-seeking behavior can be affected by such simple things as casual comments and nonverbal behaviors directed toward learners.

- A primary goal must be to aim for understanding that allows for transfer of information in a variety of circumstances.

- Dewey's ideas on differences between providing knowledge and forming ideas are relevant to educators today.

- Various teaching techniques lend themselves to promoting knowledge processing.

- Encouraging students and clinicians to imagine themselves teaching patients to think and learn is helpful in developing new skills.

- Clinicians are encouraged to practice what Schon calls reflection in action to promote thinking for today's ever-changing practice world.

- Reflecting on the differences between teaching and learning is helpful in gaining a new perspective on how to improve thinking.

References

Angelo, T. A. & Cross, K. P. (1993). *Classroom assessment techniques: A handbook for college teachers*, 2nd ed. San Francisco: Jossey-Bass.

Bargagliotti, T., Luttrell, M., & Lenburg, C. (1999, Sept. 30). Reducing threats to the implementation of a competency-based performance assessment system. *Online Journal of Issues in Nursing.* Retrieved May 25, 2004, from http://www.nursingworld.org/ojin/topic10_5.htm.

Barr, R. B. & Tagg, J. (1995). From teaching to learning: A new paradigm for undergraduate education. *Change, 27*(6), 13–25.

Benner, P. (1984). *From novice to expert: Power and excellence in nursing practice.* Menlo Park, CA: Addison-Wesley.

Billings, D. M. & Halstead, J. A. (2005). *Teaching in nursing: A guide for faculty*, 2nd ed. Philadelphia, PA: Elsevier.

Binder, F. M. (2000). So you want to be a college president? Retrieved June 3, 2004, from http://www.cosmos-club.org/journals/2000/binder.

Carkhuff, M. H. (1996). Reflective learning: Work groups as learning groups. *The Journal of Continuing Education in Nursing, 27*, 209–214.

Dewey, J. (1966). *Democracy and Education.* New York: The Free Press (Original work published 1916, Macmillan Company).

Estabrooks, C. A. (2003). Translating research into practice: Implications for organizations and administrators. *Canadian Journal of Nursing Research, 35*(3), 53–68.

Freire, P. (1998). *Pedagogy of freedom: Ethics, democracy, and civic courage.* (P. Clarke, Trans.) Lanham, MD: Rowman & Littlefield.

Institute of Medicine (IOM) (2001). *Crossing the quality chasm: A new health system for the 21st century.* Washington, DC: National Academies Press.

Institute of Medicine (IOM) (2003). *Health professions education: A bridge to quality.* Washington, DC: National Academies Press.

Perry, W. G. (1970). *Forms of intellectual and ethical development in the college years.* New York: Holt, Rinehart & Winston.

Rideout, W. (2001). *Transforming nursing education through problem-based learning.* Boston: Jones and Bartlett.

Schon, D. A. (1983). *The reflective practitioner: How professionals think in action.* New York: Basic Books.

Watkins, K. E. & Marsick, V. J. (1993). *Sculpting the learning organization: Lessons in the art and science of systemic change.* San Francisco: Jossey-Bass.

Wiggins, G. & McTighe, J. (1998). *Understanding by design.* Upper Saddle River, NJ: Merrill Prentice Hall.

CHAPTER 6

Critical Thinking and Patient-Centered Care

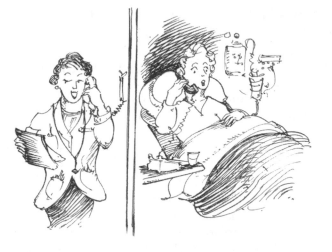

'OH... MS. McGREGOR LOOKS GOOD. HER BLOOD PRESSURE IS DOWN AND SHE'LL BE DISCHARGED IN A DAY OR TWO!'

Perhaps you heard the joke that went around before strict patient privacy laws were instituted? It goes something like this: One night the nurse on the 600 unit gets a phone call from somebody asking about Mary McGregor. The nurse grabs the chart and says, "Oh, Ms. McGregor looks good. Her blood pressure is down and she'll be discharged in a day or two!" The caller replies with obvious glee, "Oh, thank you." The nurse asks, "Are you a relative?" to which the caller replies, "No, I'm Mary McGregor and I haven't been able to get anyone to tell me anything about how I'm doing." Funny as it is, if the Institute of Medicine gets its way, no one will be able to relate to that joke because it will be so preposterous.

Providing patient-centered care has been defined by IOM as being able to "identify, respect, and care about patients' differences, values, preferences, and expressed needs; relieve pain and suffering; coordinate continuous care;

listen to, clearly inform, communicate with, and educate patients; *share deci-sion making* [italics added] and management; and continuously advocate dis-ease prevention, wellness, and promotion of healthy lifestyles, including a focus on population health." (2003, p. 4) The italicized words highlight how nurses' critical thinking interfaces with patients' CT. In this chapter we'll focus on the *thinking* involved in patient-centered care. But, first, let's consider circum-stances that probably instigated our joke. And we'll look at the state of provider–patient relationships and why this IOM competency is so important. For providers who have not yet made this paradigm shift, patient-centered care will require a drastic modification in their thinking about the relationship between patients and providers.

CHANGING PATIENT–PROVIDER RELATIONSHIPS

Let's take a look at that traditional patient–provider relationship. What decisions have you made about your health issues? Have you ever had a health provider dismiss you when you offered what you thought was a reasonable solution to your health problem? Worse yet, have you had a provider remind you that he knows better and that you should do what you're told? How did you feel? Angry? Stupid? Inept? Devalued? All of the above? This scenario exemplifies the all-powerful and disrespectful healthcare provider. And, until confronted with their behavior, most healthcare providers who behave this way are usually oblivious to other options for provider–patient relationships.

If the IOM vision becomes a reality, healthcare professionals and patients will work in partnerships. In this new relationship they will respect each other for having different, but valuable, knowledge. In the IOM version of patient-centered care, patients will no longer tolerate the traditional relationship. They will expect care tailored to their individual needs. Providers, in turn, will expect patients to do sophisticated research on the Internet, to think through their health situations, and to come up with conclusions and questions they will expect to have considered. Gone will be the days when health providers are viewed as all-knowing.

Patient-centered care is not just an IOM concept. Under a variety of other terms, such as partnerships (Enehaug, 2000), "informative relations" (Benbas-sat, Pilpel, & Tidhar, 1998), "relationship-centered care" (Nolan, Davies, Brown, Keady, & Nolan, 2004) and "person-centered care" (McCormack, 2004), this movement has been studied from moral/ethical perspectives (Hewitt-Taylor, 2003), a "consumer specialist" focus (Calabretta, 2002), and as service partner-ships (Buch & Edgren, 2001). In spite of the differences in nomenclature and focus, the underlying messages are quite similar. In Box 6.1, we've compiled some examples of patient-centered care descriptors we've found. Although

---

Box 6.1

Examples of Descriptors of Patient-Centered Care
(Sources: Buch & Edgren, 2001; Calabretta, 2002; Enehaug, 2000;
Hewitt-Taylor, 2003; McCormack, 2004; Nolan et al., 2004)

- Balance of power between provider and patient
- Empowerment of patients
- Focus on interpersonal relationships
- Shared decisions
- Understanding others' perspectives
- Common goals
- Patient autonomy promoted
- Mutual respect for each other's expertise
- Negotiation
- Acknowledgment of provider as not having all the knowledge
- Discussions of uncertainty are OK
- Patient responsibility for health
- Open communication and information exchange
- Consumer control over information

---

there are many more phrases, these should give you a snapshot of what patient-centered care looks like.

Where does your experience fit in terms of the descriptors shown in the box? Are you more familiar with the old-fashioned paternalistic provider relationships, or are these examples part of your experience? If it's the latter you recognize the wisdom of the IOM's vision. One thing we know for sure is this: This alternative to traditional approaches will affect and be affected by the thinking of both providers and patients.

PATIENT-CENTERED CARE AND CT

Patient-centered care acknowledges and celebrates patients as critical thinkers. This may be a shift in perception for many. Nurses and other providers need to consider not just their CT, but how their thinking interfaces with patients' CT. Because most patients have one or more family members and significant others who actively participate in their healthcare decision making, the actual group of affected thinkers can get fairly large. In Chapter 7 we will discuss interdisciplinary teams, and there you will see that nurses, patients, and significant others are all part of the sizable thinking/decision-making team. In the IOM's ideal healthcare delivery world, everyone's thinking would "merge" to find resolutions to the issues at hand. Figure 6.1 depicts this model of thinking through a patient's healthcare issue.

Those thinking "clouds" should merge naturally but, in fact, this doesn't happen automatically. We have a long history of viewing health providers as experts to whom patients must defer. Many older patients, especially, still have that deferential attitude. However, that patient–provider relationship is changing rapidly. Patients of all generations can access vast amounts of health information today. With implementation of patient-centered care, providers will be more likely to acknowledge and value patients' knowledge and collaborate with them in addressing health issues. However, providers cannot yet assume that patients have a certain level of knowledge, even though so much information is out there. For one thing, consumer health informatics is a burgeoning field, but it is not without its drawbacks, not the least of which is the undependable quality of the knowledge now available (Eysenbach & Jadad, 2001). Therefore, providers will need to assess patients' knowledge much more critically in the future (Coulter, Entwistle, & Gilbert, 1999). (We will examine this problem in Chapter 9 in our discussion of healthcare informatics.) Our challenge for now is threefold. We must 1) assess the patient's readiness, willingness, and ability to participate in

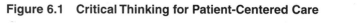

Figure 6.1   Critical Thinking for Patient-Centered Care

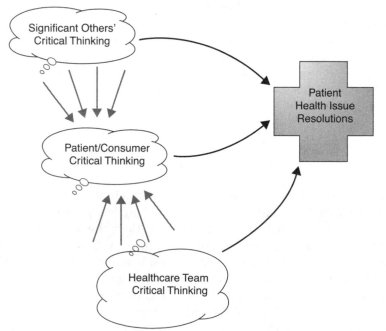

the healthcare thinking process; 2) help those patients with the actual process of thinking about their own healthcare; and 3) merge our thinking and the patient's thinking to create a mutually satisfying and functional process.

ASSESSING PATIENT READINESS, WILLINGNESS, AND ABILITY TO PARTICIPATE IN CT

Perhaps 50 years from now all patients will be accustomed to ready access to information (and the standards to judge its quality) and self-diagnostic kits. But we're not there yet. Some patients might be uncomfortable with what they see as the extra burden of being full participants in healthcare decision making; others might be dissatisfied that they are not included in the thinking process. For now, we need some way to estimate how engaged a patient is and to track potential growth in that engagement. For that we can look at CT habits of the mind.

Keeping in mind that habits of the mind are dynamic states and reflect one's penchant for CT, we could use a checklist to rate patients' thinking tendencies. Of course, we have to remember these habits vary with circumstances such as pain level and other stressors. Assessing habits of the mind is different from assessing the patient's actual skills at thinking (which we will address later); habits of the mind focus more on readiness and willingness. Look at the checklist in Box 6.2 and think about how you might use such a checklist in your practice. Even if you don't specifically rate patients' thinking habits of the mind, asking yourself these questions about each patient will help you focus on the patient as a thinking person and not some blank slate on which you and the team "do" things.

TACTICS 6.1: Reflect on Your Patients' Habits of the Mind

Clinicians and Educators

Think back to a patient encounter you (or, for educators, your student) had recently. Use the checklist in Box 6.2 to rate that patient. Then think: How did it feel to rate the patient? Can you see how such a rating might be valuable? Did it help you consider your patient in a different light?

Discussion

If you have patients who rate very low on this scale, there are several possible reasons. We must keep our expectations in context. First, consider the magnitude of the physical and emotional stress experienced in the current health situation. Pain and anxiety can be powerful in overriding natural

---

Box 6.2

CT Habits of the Mind Patient-Rating Checklist

Insert your patient's name in the blank for each item. Rate each habit of the mind as *1* (no), *2* (maybe), or *3* (yes) and mark this in the box. Remember that circumstances can change these scores, so use this information to assess where your patient is today. If your patient scores between 10 and 15, s/he is probably less likely to be an active team thinker; between 16 and 21, s/he is probably a moderately active team thinker; between 22 and 30, s/he is a very active team thinker.

☐ *Confidence:* Does _____ seem sure of himself/herself in thinking through this situation?

☐ *Contextual Perspective:* Is _____ thinking of the whole picture?

☐ *Creativity:* Is _____ likely to adapt to the situation with plans not immediately obvious to us?

☐ *Flexibility:* Is _____ able to adapt his/her thinking to this health situation?

☐ *Inquisitiveness:* Will _____ seek out information on his/her own?

☐ *Intellectual Integrity:* Will _____ consider the truth about this situation even if it goes against his/her hopes and wishes?

☐ *Intuition:* Is _____ likely to respond at a "gut level"?

☐ *Open-mindedness:* Will _____ choose the best path toward health even if it means changing his/her behavior?

☐ *Perseverance:* Will _____ hang in there and work this through?

☐ *Reflection:* Is _____ someone who stops to think back on things?

☐ **Total Score**

---

thinking habits of the mind. Second, there may be cognitive deficits because of conditions such as dementia, delirium, or neurological disease. While not considered "cognitive deficits" per se, the patient's educational level may affect thinking. In these cases, don't forget those patients' significant others as thinking team members; complete the checklist with them in mind. Third, cultural or generational issues might cause a patient to think it disrespectful to openly participate in health issue thinking. (We discussed some of these ideas in Chapter 3). In those cases, it is our responsibility to let those people know that it is not only OK, but desirable, to think along with us.

HELPING PATIENTS WITH THEIR THINKING PROCESSES

Once we have a feel for patients' CT tendencies, we can better gauge how much encouragement, if any, they need to exercise their thinking skills alongside ours. In other words, for patients and significant others we need to determine what's in those thinking "clouds" shown in Figure 6.1 on p. 98. To help you focus on their thinking let's look at each of the seven CT skills, explore how patients use those skills, and consider what we can do to promote them. We have addressed the skills in alphabetical order; this does not imply any ranking of their importance.

Analyzing

Separating or breaking a whole into parts to discover their nature, function, and relationships. Can you imagine patients breaking down options for their care, such as for treatment of diabetes? Of course you can. Studying the pros and cons of insulin therapy and oral hypoglycemics is an analytical process. Helping patients analyze the complexities of a diabetic diet helps them follow recommendations. It's not enough to hand dietary guidelines to patients; they need to break that down into something that translates into their breakfast, lunch, dinner, snacks, grocery lists, restaurant options, vacation diets, sick days, and so on. Coulter et al. (1999), using focus groups, found that patients were dissatisfied with the information they got from healthcare providers. They wanted a full range of treatment options and to learn the pros and cons of each. They wanted materials to help them feel knowledgeable enough to participate equally in decision making. They didn't want simplistic conclusions; they wanted empowerment through knowledge. If providers and patients together analyze situations—break things down to essential information—they will better understand which options are appropriate and make more informed decisions. Patients then will be more likely to adhere to treatments such as dietary changes and their care will be more centered on them because it will be more consistent with their lifestyle.

Applying Standards

Judging according to established personal, professional, or social rules or criteria. This is an interesting cognitive skill. It is closely aligned with what one values. In a recent class exercise we asked RN/BSN students to share personal standards they applied in their practices. Here are some of their answers: "I always check to see if my patients need pain medication right at the end of my shift and I remind them that staff will be in transition for the next hour. I don't want them sitting there waiting for pain medication." "I always talk about what I'm doing while I'm doing tasks in patients' rooms." "I try to teach something every time I'm in the room." "I always ask patients, 'How can I help you today?' " Aren't those wonderful standards?

Now, let's think about patients' standards. How often do we ask patients what they expect of us? What is their definition of standard of care and might those standards be in conflict with ours? Healthcare providers are apt to forget that patients don't know the usual routines that are taken for granted in healthcare. Patients might expect all nurses to ask about pain medication at the end of the shift, as the nurse above did. If the nurse on the next shift doesn't, patients are apt to think that she isn't doing her job.

Think about the patient who is constantly pressing his call light for seemingly trivial reasons. Might that patient think this is the expected standard of nursing care on an evening shift on a medical floor? People often think of nurses as being like waiters—you just call them when you want something. Rather than getting frustrated with patients like this, we can try to educate them about the norms and standards of care and ask them what they expect as routines.

A common example of conflicting standards is the patient who is angry at having to wait in the office 45 minutes for their physician or nurse practitioner. They obviously have an expectation that a 3 p.m. appointment means that they'll be seen within five minutes or so—as they do at the hairdresser, for example. Sometimes a straightforward explanation of what life is like in a medical office—people have unexpected needs that disrupt schedules—is enough to help a patient develop a more realistic standard and expectation of care. Patients *and* providers must have a full knowledge of how the system works for a true partnership to exist (Enehaug, 2000).

Another consideration concerning *applying standards* is linked to patient access to information. Patients not only read about healthcare issues in magazines, they can, for example, go online and retrieve the same guidelines for diabetes management that their health provider is using. In line with that diabetes management example, the National Institutes of Health web site (http:// betterdiabetescare.nih.gov) cites seven dimensions of patient-centered care, including respect; information and communication; and coordination and integration of care (*Better Diabetes Care*, n.d.). This site promotes a true partnership between patients with diabetes and their providers. Today's patients who use the thinking skill of applying standards will keep us on our toes. If we focus only on our application of standards, without considering the patients' application of those same standards, we will create conflict, waste time, and diminish patient-centered care.

Discriminating

Recognizing differences and similarities among things or situations and distinguishing carefully as to category or rank. We wouldn't think of this as a cognitive skill that we readily identify from patients' perspectives. After all, we see distinguishing the finer points in healthcare situations as requiring our expert eyes, ears, and intuition. However, when we consider patients' abilities to make fine distinctions about their bodies, we can appreciate their ability to discriminate.

Pain assessment, for example, requires patient discrimination. Consider the question, "On a scale of zero to 10, with 10 being your worst pain, what number do you rank your pain at now?" The answer requires mighty powers of discrimination, with potentially dire consequences (often unrealized by patients). Nurses decide between Tylenol and Vicodin based on those numbers! Should we pay more mind to how well patients are able to discriminate when we ask that question? And we must not let our own biases invade. Imagine the scenario going through this nurse's mind as she asks a patient to rate pain: "This patient ranks her pain at a 3 on the 1–10 scale. She is a woman so the worst pain she's had is probably childbirth. I had a baby so I have a good idea of what her 3 would be. OK, so she's in reasonable pain." But, what if this woman suffers from migraine or cluster headaches? She may be using that pain as her standard.

The point is, the number is minimally relevant unless we can relate it to a baseline. The number only allows for accurate *discrimination* when the patient shares what the pain compares to. We must ask about that comparison to find out how the patient is making the distinction between, say, a 5 and a 3. Patient-centered care depends on understanding the patient's unique perspective, thinking, and discriminating skills.

Calabretta (2002) went so far as to call patients "consumer specialists" because of this acute self-discriminating ability relative to their health. "Because patients can afford to focus narrowly on their own concerns, learning only about their condition, they have the possibility of ultimately becoming 'consumer specialists.' In addition, all patients have the inherent knowledge of their own symptoms and the experience of living with a disease that physicians lack" (p. 33).

Information Seeking

Searching for evidence, facts, or knowledge by identifying relevant sources and gathering objective, subjective, historical, and current data from those sources. In today's world of easy access to information, patients can and will access information with or without our help. They can, for example, go to the American Diabetes Association web site, pull up the section for healthcare professionals, and read the recommendations for care. Increasingly, we find patients doing just that. They read self-help books, magazine articles, and view TV shows, all of which provide information. While some patients are able to do extensive research on their health issues all on their own, others could and might do that if healthcare providers guided them by identifying resources such as web sites, patient-information libraries, and self-help books.

Our role as providers must be that of coaching patients to be seekers of information and we must help them evaluate which sources of information are legitimate. We are well past the days when our role in patients' information-seeking is to merely hand them brochures. We now need to be partners in seeking information. We must listen to and value what our patients find, and respond, not in a dismissive manner, but using a collegial model of deciding together the value of that information. Sharing and valuing each other's information promote patient-centered care.

As we have mentioned earlier and will discuss in Chapter 9, the issue of judging information, especially that found on the Internet, is still problematic. Some organizations are working diligently to improve this situation and develop instruments to judge the quality of web site information. (We list some in Chapter 9.) Unfortunately, we have a long way to go before these instruments are consistently validated. Gagliardi and Jadad (2002) found 51 new web site rating instruments; only five had information allowing them to be evaluated and none of those had been validated. They questioned the value of these incompletely developed instruments, asking: "Is it desirable or necessary to assess the quality of health information on the [i]nternet? If so, is it an achievable goal given that quality is a construct for which we have no gold standard?" (p. 571). Until these questions are answered, we must use our CT and help patients use their CT to choose the best sources of information and evaluate the quality of that information. The folks at Vanderbilt University have an interesting system to help patients get the best information. Their Medical Center and Eskind Biomedical Library have developed a Patient Informatics Consult Service, which gives patients information prescriptions they can take to librarians who then collect the information and create a report that is delivered to the clinician and patient (Williams, Gish, Giuse, Sathe, & Carrell, 2001). Now that's CT *creativity* at work!

Logical Reasoning

Drawing inferences or conclusions that are supported in or justified by evidence. This cognitive skill is used by everyone to some degree. Most patients today will not accept pat answers that aren't supported by the evidence of their symptoms. They will, and should, question these answers. On the other hand, we can also point out to patients that there is much we still don't know—that we don't have evidence for some things. "Healthcare professionals should acknowledge that they do not possess complete and irrefutable knowledge . . . [and] enter into discussions with patients in which uncertainties and conflicting views can be explored openly" (Hewitt-Taylor, 2003, p. 1327). Working together with patients using available information, however incomplete it might be, we can help patients draw conclusions that are easier to accept because they can see the logic behind them.

Consider this case study: Mrs. Jones is 75; she has a diagnosis of diverticulosis and colonic stricture; she has been suffering from diarrhea since finishing one course of antibiotics for a recent urinary tract infection. Based on her physical exam findings, she was placed on metronidazole to cover both clostridium difficile colitis and diverticulitis. When she sees her nurse practitioner (NP) on a follow-up visit, she states that she has stopped taking the metronidazole because it made her nauseated and she didn't like the taste it left in her mouth. When the NP said she needed a referral to GI and an abdominal CT, Mrs. Jones replied, "I don't like that doctor and I'm not having another CT." Continuing to ask for something to help stop the diarrhea, but refusing all suggestions, the patient was a challenge to the NP, who was struggling alone with the logical reasoning. Totally frustrated, she finally laid all the facts in front of the patient, including ways to disguise the taste of the pill, and said, "Here are the only conclusions I can make with these facts. Do you see a different conclusion here?" The patient replied, "Oh, I thought there were other things I could do, but I see that these are my choices."

Initially, this passive patient wanted the nurse to draw all the conclusions and make the decisions. Ultimately, however, when presented with the facts and given the option to draw her own conclusion, the patient engaged her logical reasoning and drew inferences based on the available evidence. (By the way, the patient reported that metronidazole and peanut butter taste great!) This situation is not unusual. Patients who see health providers as all-knowing don't engage in the decision making, but wait passively until a conclusion is passed down. Patients often can state what they don't want, outside of the context of all possible choices. When faced with making decisions themselves or in partnership with providers, they can see the logic used by the provider, and add their own logical reasoning.

Predicting

Envisioning a plan and its consequences. Patients may be better at the cognitive skill of predicting than healthcare providers; they can see how their lives will change by the health issue at hand. A good question to help patients use this skill, for example, is "Knowing that diabetes is a progressive condition (meaning that you will likely need more medications over time), how do you see yourself dealing with this over the next few years?" This question helps patients think about the future and increases the chances that they will recognize the consequences of their decisions. It is important for providers to help patients see alternative "right" answers. There may be good, better, and best options, or even three "betters" and two "bests."

Helping patients with predictive thinking is valuable because patients know themselves, and the circumstances of their daily lives, best. Predicting is especially important when patients are first faced with a chronic illness that will change their lifestyles. The process of predicting helps them internalize their new health situation and accept their realities; it is one road on the journey through the normal grief stages of anger, blaming someone for the situation, and denial that occur with any lifestyle change. Predicting consequences may not come naturally to some and can be culturally based as well as dependent on cognitive and developmental skills. Our job as providers is to facilitate opportunities for patients to use this skill to promote patient-centered care.

Predictive thinking, so important in dealing with chronic illness, is a driving force behind the shift away from provider-centered care, a paradigm for acute illness management (*Better Diabetes Care*, n.d.). In the case of an acute illness, the provider takes more control, but with chronic illness management, once the patient is out the hospital or office door, he is the one in control. Predictive thinking about what's outside that door must be the result of a partnership between patients and providers.

Transforming Knowledge

Patients probably have to *transform knowledge (change or convert the condition, nature, form, or function of concepts among contexts)* more than their providers. Patients with this skill use information to take control of new health situations. Consider patient education: you know that you need to impart medical knowledge in a way that patients can understand it. Among the most successful knowledge-transformation examples are consumer self-help groups, which allow patients with similar conditions to talk to each other, teach each other, and translate medical lingo into something they can learn from.

It behooves healthcare providers to think about how they can learn from consumer groups. Some primary care settings have done this by having group appointments for patients with similar conditions, such as diabetes or pregnancy. The provider saves time by not having to repeat things and patients benefit by receiving information from both the provider and others in similar situations. Group interactions are great facilitators for transforming knowledge. Transforming the provider's knowledge into the patient's reality, and vice versa, provides increased opportunities for patient-centered care.

HOW TO MERGE OUR THINKING WITH PATIENT THINKING

With this perspective of how patients can and do use their thinking skills, what can educators and clinicians do to make this team thinking the norm?

Patient-centered care does not happen automatically. Even though it seems a ludicrous statement, it is easy to forget the patient as we go along our way as healthcare providers. The first job, then, is to *remember the patient*. The second is to validate, validate, validate our conclusions with the patient. The third job is to coax and coach patient thinking.

Remember the Patient

In our nursing classes, when we get to the part about drawing conclusions—such as nursing diagnoses—we often ask our students, "Now that you've concluded that there is a problem needing nursing care, what will your next step be?" The typical response (based on their familiarity with the assessing, planning, implementing, and evaluating phases of the nursing process) is, "Start planning." The answer we are looking for, however, is "Validate that conclusion with the patient." In all our years of teaching, neither of us has ever gotten that response without prompting. And that's even with our teaching patient-centered care from the get-go. Why is it so easy to "forget the patient" when we keep saying we value patient-centered care?

Here's an example. A student caring for a patient whose wife had died four months earlier made a nursing diagnosis of dysfunctional grieving based on evidence that the patient could not speak of his wife without crying. That student, with the teacher's prompting, sought the patient's validation of that conclusion by asking, "Mr. Jones, based on my assessment, I'm thinking that my nursing diagnosis is dysfunctional grieving. What do you think?" Mr. Jones was quick to put the student in her place. "I am grieving, but there's nothing dysfunctional about crying over my wonderful wife who left me only four months ago!" In response, this student changed her diagnosis to *incomplete* grieving, even though the NANDA (2003) classification has no such label (and still doesn't—it has *anticipatory* and *dysfunctional grieving* only). There wasn't a problem—just a conclusion, based on facts, made jointly with the patient. This is a pure example of logical reasoning and in this case the patient's logical reasoning was better than the student's. She was more focused, initially, on following context-free rules—a common occurrence with novice-level thinking. But she was able, with the patient's partnership, to demonstrate *logical reasoning* and *transforming knowledge*.

Validate, Validate, Validate

The process of validation cannot be overemphasized. Think about your practice; how often do you solicit patients' validation to see if your thinking is on track? How often do you validate with yourself that you are valuing the

---

Box 6.3

Validation Remarks to Promote Patient Participation in Decisions

- Here's what I think; do you agree?
- What would you say is going on here?
- How is all of this affecting you?
- Does it seem that way to you? It does to me.
- Let's think about this together for a minute.
- Only you know your daily living situation.
- Can we find a way through this together?
- Let me explain my thinking to you.
- What do you think?
- Does this feel OK?
- Do you agree with this?
- This is what I'm thinking; what do you think?
- I'm interested in your take on all of this.
- If you could change this, what would be different?
- If you had a magic wand, what would you have it do?

---

patient's part in the thinking process? See Box 6.3 for examples of remarks that support both kinds of validation.

TACTICS 6.2: Reflect on Your Validation Remarks

Clinicians

Carry a copy of the validation remarks in Box 6.3 in your pocket for a couple days as you work with patients. Periodically, pull it out and check off which comments you've made. At the end of each day, look at how many comments you've made.

Educators

Distribute a copy of Box 6.3 to your students and ask them to track how many times they make such remarks over the course of a day or two when working with patients. You might also think about how many of these comments you use with students to validate your thinking with them.

Discussion

These remarks may seem simple, but many important things we do as nurses *are* simple. Remember the old adage: "for want of a nail the shoe is lost, for want of a shoe the horse is lost, for want of a horse the rider is lost." There's a lot of truth to that; don't forget the simple things, they have huge consequences. Simple can be powerful.

Buch and Edgren (2001) suggested that patients be interviewed soon after admission to the hospital to "explore expectations, needs and demands" (p. 69). Doing that would set the stage for thinking partnerships at the outset of the patient–provider encounter. The patient would expect to be a partner in decision making, either as a direct participant or by validating conclusions.

Coaxing and Coaching Patient Thinking

Most patients respect healthcare providers; they don't want to step on their toes and don't want to take up their time. Most patients are also reluctant to push for team thinking if their providers don't indicate that this is desirable. Using the validation remarks listed in Box 6.3 might help providers encourage patient participation, but there's more to it than that. We must do more than just verbally validate our thinking with them; we have to personify openness to their thinking and show them that we value them as people, not only as patients. That's a tough one to put in a box—it's linked to our personal interaction styles and requires subtle nonverbal communication. We asked some nurses how they show patients they are open to "sitting down and thinking" together. Box 6.4 lists ideas those nurses shared. Add your unique ideas to this list.

ARE THERE NEGATIVES TO PATIENT-CENTERED CARE?

Clearly, we value patient-centered care, but are there negatives to this? Certainly. Two of the biggest are time and power. It takes more time to practice true patient-centered care—or so it would seem on the face of it. As providers we have to give up power and share it with patients and, if we consider that honestly, that makes us feel vulnerable. It's hard to admit that we don't have all the control or all the answers.

Time

Let's look at time. Say you have a passive patient who doesn't push to get involved in decisions. What do you do? You probably answer, "Get the patient involved, of course." Now, picture yourself on a particularly busy medical unit and ask yourself what you'd do. If you're like most, you'd be happy that the patient is not slowing you down, asking questions and expressing opinions on how things should be done. This is our reality; we're busy people and practic-

---

Box 6.4

Strategies to Help Healthcare Providers Encourage Patient Participation in the Thinking Process

- Stay in the room, don't talk to them from the doorway.
- Pay attention to your body language and to theirs.
- Sit down so you're at eye level with them.
- Use open questions and comments, such as *Tell me about* . . . instead of closed questions, which imply that you expect a short answer.
- Touch them, but be respectful of their space and cultural norms.
- Use collaborative thinking language such as "We should think this through." "Let's look at some possible conclusions." "Can we analyze this together?"
- Use phrases that let them know that their situation is not so unique that they can't discuss it; for example, *Some people feel anxious when* . . .
- Address them respectfully; find out if they prefer *Mr.* or *Mrs.* or *Professor, Reverend*, and so on.
- Don't look at your watch, no matter how busy you are.
- Be direct and honest; for example, tell them when the schedule is backed up and why.
- If you feel like avoiding that patient, reflect on why you feel that way.

---

ing patient-centered care can be very time-consuming. That's probably the real reason why it's not the norm.

We ask you to reconsider this assumption. Does patient-centered care really take more time in the long run or does it seem that way in the short run? How much time do we spend doing things that *we* decide are best for the patients only to find that those patients have no investment in our ideas because they weren't involved in the decisions? How many extra trips down the hall do we have to make because our patients feel isolated and at the mercy of all those providers who are making decisions *for* them? What is the price of making our patients feel powerless?

Power

Now, let's look at power—ours and patients'. According to the IOM (2003), "the patient is the source of control" (p. 47) and providers must "allow patients to have unfettered access to the information contained in their medical records" (p. 52). Are you old enough to remember the days when it was unheard of to show a patient his chart? Do you work in a setting where patients who ask to look at their charts are still put off: "You'll need to wait until the doctor can sit down with you." When we were students we were usually taught phrases to use when patients asked us what their blood pressure was: "It's just fine, don't worry about it; it's a little high but it's fine." What nonsense that seems now with the new focus on patient-centered care! Some of you might be saying, "Gee, that's still done on our unit!" We hope not, but we wouldn't be surprised.

Don't you wonder why we kept patients' health information secret from them? We think some of it had to do with a misplaced sense of power, as well as a desire to protect patients and ourselves. Perhaps it was predicated on a fear of litigation, which is certainly a consideration in the United States. Traditionally, we are the burden-carriers *for* patients. We know what's best for them. At the same time, we keep their identities as people separated from our identities; otherwise we might spend too much time worrying about what it would be like to be in their situation. We want to distance ourselves from the horror of being sick. You can probably think of other reasons to keep your distance, too.

Oops, it's time for therapy again. Maybe it's time that educators help students deal with their mortality as a way to promote patient-centered care. That's not such a far-fetched idea. If we can help providers see how similar they are to patients, right at the start of their education, instead of making them feel superior to and separate from them, then we will minimize the power issues that interfere with patient-centered care.

We need to accept that we are not there to protect patients from the truth—that healthcare is a collaborative process. Providers are supposed to help patients think through health issues with open eyes. Hickson et al. (2002) studied patient complaints and malpractice risk; their results were consistent with earlier similar studies. "Patients who saw physicians with the highest numbers of lawsuits were more likely to complain that their physicians would not listen or return telephone calls, were rude, and did not show respect" (p. 2955). While fear of litigation should not be a primary force driving patient-centered care, it can serve as a reminder that we want to avoid adversarial relationships and we want patients in the loop in the decision-making process. In the long run, withholding information is not protection—it's simply not good practice.

PAUSE AND PONDER: WHERE IS THE BALANCE?

What else can educators and clinicians do? We will leave this question for you to ponder. Keep in mind that there are no easy answers to these complex issues. We'll bet every reader can think of a patient who was so controlling that the only solution seemed to be saying, "Could you just listen to me and do as I ask?" Such negative situations always seem to stand out more than the positive ones. We've also had many patients who reached wonderful "aha" points after collaborative problem solving. There will, of course, always be extremes that challenge our commitment to patient-centered care.

One useful guideline to remember is balance. Ideal patient-centered care is a balance of patient thinking and provider thinking within the realities of each situation. Many factors—knowledge, access to knowledge, overt and covert permission to think, cultural beliefs about roles, habits of the mind and thinking skills, power and control—affect thinking and patient-centered care. Our job is to keep thinking in spite of time constraints, taking advantage of our CT and that of our patients.

Reflection Cues

- Patient-centered care, as envisioned by the IOM, must include a focus on patient and provider thinking.

- Traditional patient–provider relationships were hierarchical, with the provider doing the thinking for the patient.

- Patient-centered care must start with a collaborative relationship.

- Patients, significant others, and the team of healthcare providers must work to merge their thinking toward one end—a healthcare issue resolution.

- Challenges for providers who want to think with patients are three-fold. We must: assess the patient's readiness, willingness, and ability to participate in the healthcare thinking process; help patients with the actual process of thinking about their own healthcare; merge our thinking and the patient's thinking to create a mutually satisfying and functional process.

- Assessing readiness, willingness, and ability to participate in collaborative thinking can be done by considering patients' CT habits of the mind, taking into account contextual factors that might affect those habits of the mind.

- Helping patients with their thinking processes can be done by focusing on each of seven CT cognitive skills.

- Patients can be encouraged to *analyze*, breaking issues down into manageable parts.

- Providers can determine patients' expectations of standards of care and share with patients their *application of standards.*

- Patients are often able to *discriminate* the nuances of their responses as well as, or better than, providers.

- Sharing *logical reasoning* processes with patients can help them see how we come to conclusions, enabling them to draw their own conclusions.

- *Predictive* thinking helps patients see the reality ahead and may help them through a grief process brought on by a change in health.

- *Transforming knowledge* is crucial to effective patient teaching; consumer groups often do very well at transforming medical knowledge into a usable form for consumers.

- Merging provider and patient thinking means remembering patients and validating conclusions with them.

- Negative aspects of patient-centered care can be seen as time and power issues.

- While patient-centered care may seem time consuming, in the long run it may save time.

- Giving up the power of the traditional hierarchical provider–patient relationship can make us feel vulnerable.

- Power issues between providers and patients may be addressed by having providers consider their own mortality.

References

Benbassat, J., Pilpel, D., & Tidhar, M. (1998). Patients' preferences for participation in clinical decision making: A review of published surveys. *Behavioral Medicine, 24*(2), *81*(8). Retrieved June 3, 2004, from http://infotrac.galegroup.com/itw/infomark/433/307/52152671w2/purl=rcl_ITOF_0_A210660.

Better diabetes care—what we want to achieve through systems changes. (n.d.) Retrieved August 3, 2004, from http://betterdiabetescare.nih.gov/WHATpatientcenteredcare.htm.

Buch, T. & Edgren, L. (2001). Patients as partners in intensive care units: A conceptual analysis of the literature. *Nursing in Critical Care, 6*(2), 64–70.

Calabretta, N. (2002). Consumer-driven, patient-centered health care in the age of electronic information. *Journal of the Medical Library Association, 90*(1), 32–37.

Coulter, A., Entwistle, V., & Gilbert, D. (1999). Sharing decisions with patients: Is the information good enough? *BMJ, 318,* 318–322.

Enehaug, I. H. (2000). Patient participation requires a change of attitude in health care. *International Journal of Health Care Quality Assurance, 13*(4), 178–181.

Eysenbach, G. & Jadad, A. R. (2001). Evidence-based patient choice and consumer health informatics in the internet age. *Journal of Medical Internet Research, 3*(2), e19. Retrieved August 3, 2004, from http://www.jmir.org/2001/2/e19/index.htm.

Gagliardi, A. & Jadad, A. R. (2002). Examination of instruments used to rate quality of health information on the internet: Chronicle of a voyage with an unclear destination. *BMJ, 324,* 560–573.

Hewitt-Taylor, J. (2003). Issues involved in promoting patient autonomy in health care. *British Journal of Nursing, 12*(22), 1323–1330.

Hickson, G. B., Federspiel, C. F., Pichert, J. W., Miller, C. S., Gauld-Jaeger, J., & Bost, P. (2002). Patient complaints and malpractice risk. *JAMA, 287,* 2951–2957.

Institute of Medicine (IOM) (2003). *Health professions education: A bridge to quality.* Washington, DC: National Academies Press.

McCormack, B. (2004). Person-centredness in gerontological nursing: An overview of the literature. *Journal of Clinical Nursing, 13*(3a), 31–38. Retrieved August 3, 2004, from CINAHL Database with Full Text database. (Document ID: 2004093693).

NANDA International (2003). *Nursing diagnoses: Definitions & classification 2003–2004.* Philadelphia: Author.

Nolan, M. R., Davies, S., Brown, J., Keady, J., & Nolan, J. (2004). Beyond "person-centred" care: A new vision for gerontological nursing. *Journal of Clinical Nursing, 13*(3a), 45–53. Retrieved August 3, 2004, from CINAHL Database with Full Text database. (Document ID: 2004093694).

Williams, M. D., Gish, K. W., Giuse, N. B., Sathe, N. A., & Carrell, D. L. (2001). The patient informatics consult service (PICS): An approach for a patient-centered service. *Bulletin of the Medical Library Association, 89*(2), 185–193.

CHAPTER 7

Critical Thinking and Interdisciplinary Teams

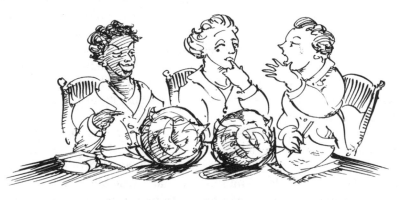

`I DON'T THINK THAT'S WHAT THEY MEANT`

"Two Heads Are Better Than One."

It's hard to imagine anyone has not heard this saying. The better outcome resulting from two or more heads thinking together is the purpose of work in interdisciplinary teams.

Participants in the Institute of Medicine (IOM) study (2003) strongly believed that combining "heads" was essential to improving healthcare, and, therefore included "work in interdisciplinary teams" as one of their five competency recommendations for practice and education. They envisioned the work of interdisciplinary teams (IDT) as the ability to, "cooperate, collaborate, communicate, and integrate care in teams to ensure that care is continuous and reliable" (p. 45). These teams are composed of members from different professions who are able to "integrate their observations, bodies of expertise, and spheres of decision making" (p. 54). This team approach is particularly important today. "Interdisciplinary teams are critical in dealing with the increasing complexity of care, coordinating and responding to multiple patient needs, keeping pace with the demands of new technology, responding to the demands of payers, and delivering care across settings" (IOM, 2003, p. 54).

The IOM did not address CT directly, but how can individuals, let alone IDT members address all the factors in the last quote without solid CT skills? Look at the language used by the IOM: "dealing with," "coordinating," "responding," "integrate their observations," "expertise," "decision making." CT is the engine that drives those activities.

We suspect the IOM was simply assuming we could see the underlying CT. But such assumptions contribute to why details of thinking are frequently overlooked in complex processes such as IDT work. When we make these basic assumptions and do not emphasize the underlying CT we make it harder to learn and teach others how to effectively achieve the IDT competency.

There are also added layers of thinking in teams and groups that must be addressed if we want IDT to be successful. Thinking as a group is not simply a collection of people giving their input. "Two heads are better than one" implies an expansion of thinking, not simple addition. IDT thinking is synergistic as each thinker builds upon the CT of others and, in turn, modifies and recontributes new thinking.

Sharing individual input and simple addition of information require limited thinking ability (Bensimon & Neumann, 1993) and are the most common forms of teamwork because of their ease. Teams of individuals from different disciplines are generally considered multidisciplinary. True interdisciplinary teams that engage in high levels of synergistic thinking require individuals who understand and appreciate both their individual thinking and thinking skills needed for system thinking or team thinking (Senge, 1990; Bensimon & Neumann, 1993).

This chapter begins with an illustration of the important links between CT and IDT thinking and a discussion of IDT yesterday and today. We then answer these questions: *How* is CT in IDT different than individual CT? *What* interferes with IDT thinking and *what* cultivates it?

LINKS BETWEEN CT AND IDT

Figure 7.1 illustrates the linkages between individual thinking and team thinking and the positive outcomes of that synergistic CT. The different disciplines participating in an IDT are represented by the heads with individual thinking clouds. Their individual CT skills merge into team thinking (TT) as they collaborate through discussion/dialogue. Discussion/dialogue, the center

Figure 7.1   Interdisciplinary Team Thinking

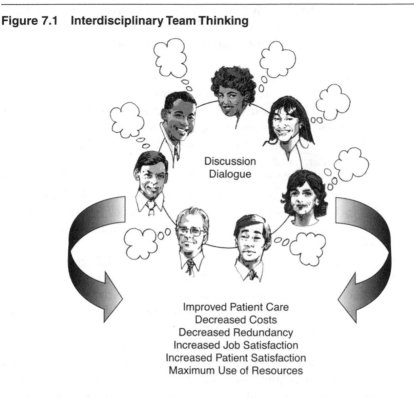

Discussion
Dialogue

Improved Patient Care
Decreased Costs
Decreased Redundancy
Increased Job Satisfaction
Increased Patient Satisfaction
Maximum Use of Resources

of the circle, is the key to true interdisciplinary team thinking because it makes the most of "two heads are better than one." Team thinking leads to at least the six positive outcomes listed below the IDT.

IDT YESTERDAY AND TODAY

IDTs are not new. Examining their history provides insight into aspects that have not been successful, helping us avoid them in the future. Clarification of IDT terminology over time helps us stay focused on true IDT thinking not demonstrated in other forms of teamwork. And, identifying current proponents of IDT helps underline both its historical and current value in healthcare.

IDT History in a Nutshell

Employing an interdisciplinary approach to work and recognizing the value of team thinking began long ago. Civilization as we know it would not have survived without the collaborative thinking of folks with different skills needed to save the clan from saber-toothed tiger attacks, harvest crops, raise barns, build factories and fly into space. We have vivid examples of team work today in the Amish culture, for example, where large tasks such as barn raising are only accomplished by teams.

Interdisciplinary teams in healthcare have a somewhat shorter history. Baldwin (1996), in an article describing the history of IDT in practice and education, traced some of the earliest healthcare teams to mission hospitals in India prior to the 1900s. These teams were composed of physicians, nurses, and "auxiliaries." London's Pioneer Health Centre in the 1920s focused on collaborative healthcare teams and a "positive health" model. The London Centre inspired similar projects in South Africa and Israel with the development of primary health teams in community-based health programs. The Montefiore Hospital in New York City began using healthcare teams of physicians, social workers and nurses in 1948. It too focused on health and illness prevention models more than medical models of care.

Baldwin (1996) also described seven phases of interdisciplinary team work in the U.S.A. Phase I began in the 1940s with federal funding and included primary care health team development through IDT education and training. Phases II and III occurred in the 1960s and 1970s, concurrent with the community mental health movement and the start of groups such as the Institute for Health Team Development. By the end of the 1970s federal funding for IDT projects had declined significantly. Phases IV and V, beginning in the early 1980s, included the Veterans Administration work on IDT training in geriatrics and a national focus on rural populations. Phase VI saw a change in funding sources, from public to private, including the Robert Woods Johnson and the Kellogg Foundations. Phase VII began in the mid 1990s with a renewed interest in the potential for IDT to enhance healthcare quality.

Throughout those phases, the IDTs are composed of many health professions (nurses, physicians, social workers, physical therapists, occupational therapists, pharmacists, recreational therapists, dentists, optometrists, osteopathic physicians, and psychologists to name the predominant professions). Baldwin alluded to thinking as a key component to success when he said, "Interdisciplinary healthcare teams are not an end in themselves, but a means for more effective communication and cooperation . . . " (1996, p. 183). Communication and cooperation are only effective with CT to back them up.

Clarification of IDT Terminology

Teams are groups of individuals with different skills and abilities working together to achieve a goal. The literature frequently interchanges the adjective preceding the word "team" to describe a group's composition. Those adjectives include "multidisciplinary," "interdisciplinary," and most recently, "interprofessional."

The term "interprofessional" was recommended by the National Academies of Practice (Simpson, et al., 2001, p. 5). In 2000 they convened a panel of 17 experts representing 11 disciplines involved in healthcare to review over 750 citations using the terminology, "interdisciplinary healthcare." The goal of the National Academies of Practice was "to promote the implementation of cost-effective interprofessional health practice that leads to better healthcare outcomes" (p. 6). They focused on three recommendations for achieving the goal: 1) disseminating information on successful models of IDT practice, 2) increasing opportunities for healthcare professionals to make referrals to each other and practice collaboratively, and 3) advocating for changes in legal and reimbursement policies to support IDT practice.

Table 7.1 below lists characteristics of "multidisciplinary," "interdisciplinary," and "interprofessional" teams. For the purposes of this chapter we will

Table 7.1   Comparison of Multidisciplinary, Interdisciplinary, and Interprofessional Teams

	Multidisciplinary Teams (adapted from Siegler, 1998)	Interdisciplinary Teams (adapted from Siegler, 1998)	Interprofessional Teams (adapted from Simpson, et al., 2001)
Membership	Professionals from a variety of disciplines	All necessary disciplines	A partnership among professionals, individuals, families, and communities
Sources of information	Members contribute information from their own area of expertise within the roles of their specific discipline	Patients and/or significant others provide information along with members of the disciplines	Patients and/or significant others, members of the disciplines related to the patient's care provide information
			(continues)

Table 7.1   Comparison of Multidisciplinary, Interdisciplinary, and Interprofessional Teams *(continued)*

	Multidisciplinary Teams (adapted from Siegler, 1998)	Interdisciplinary Teams (adapted from Siegler, 1998)	Interprofessional Teams (adapted from Simpson, et al., 2001)
Leadership	Leadership and membership are fixed	Leadership and membership vary depending on the situation	Leadership is based on expertise that matches the situation
Decision making	One person makes the final treatment decisions	All members work together to come up with both alternative solutions and final decisions.	A shared responsibility for decision making and problem solving
Focus of Care	Task orientation	Collaboration to see the bigger picture	A shared biopsychosocial paradigm

use the term "interdisciplinary" as it is the most commonly used, but define it more comprehensively with characteristics of "interdisciplinary" and "interprofessional" teams as identified in Table 7.1.

Based on the above descriptions it may be difficult to make clean distinctions among these teams in the real world of healthcare which has no neat boxes as book chapters do. In practice there are hybrids of these teams. The predominant form of teamwork and thinking found in healthcare today matches the "multidisciplinary" column as demonstrated in the scenario that follows.

Team Thinking in Practice

To illustrate the application of team thinking in practice we created a TACTICS to encourage your CT.

TACTICS 7.1: Practice Setting Team Meeting and Thinking

1. Read Scenario 7.1 below
2. Find the thinking that occurred.
3. Identify the thinking done by the individuals by comparing the scenario descriptions with the CT vocabulary on your 17 dimensions card.
4. Compare the events with the characteristics of the different kinds of teams in Table 7.1.
5. Make a list of what you would do to make the team more interdisciplinary and, to yourself or with a colleague, explain the CT needed to do it more effectively.
6. Think about the kind of thinking that may have occurred beyond individual thinking. This last task is challenging at this point in the chapter because we have not yet begun a discussion of team thinking, but all good thinkers enjoy a challenge, so see how you do.

Scenario 7.1

Practice Setting Team Meeting and Thinking

CD is a 75-year-old married male admitted to a sub-acute unit for rehabilitation following a mild right sided ischemic stroke (CVA), attributed to atrial fibrillation, which has affected his left side. He agreed to a short stay to improve his strength and functional abilities. Medications were adjusted prior to discharge from the hospital. Now, a week later, he is participating in the care conference which includes his physical therapist (PT), occupational therapist (OT), speech and language pathologist (SLP), his primary nurse (RN), registered dietician (RD), physician (MD), social worker (SW) and charge nurse. Fortunately his regular doctor and nurse practitioner are on staff and round at this facility regularly. No other family members are present. He says "I want to go home tomorrow. I am really feeling good and I don't see any sense in wasting everyone's time."

Going home has been a recurrent theme since he arrived. The SW has done his evaluation, learning that CD is the primary caregiver to his wife who has dementia and is being cared for by their son who flew in when CD was hospitalized. The SW reports that CD is a retired engineer with good insurance benefits.

PT, OT and SLP all report that CD has made great progress this past week. He is ambulating 50 feet with contact guard. He is "a bit" impulsive in his movements and decision making; he needs frequent cues to attend to tasks at hand. He makes his needs known.

*They believe he could benefit from at least 2 more weeks of ther-
apy, twice daily, for safety and strength reasons. SLP says that his
swallowing problems are also improving and he has advanced to a
Dysphagia II diet. He continues to take his meals in his room to
avoid distraction, maintaining aspiration precautions. He eats
impulsively, gulping and not chewing his food completely. The RD
tells the group that CD's weight has been stable and his nutritional
needs are being met based on a completed calorie count.*

*The RN identified the following problems: Impaired physical
mobility, Toileting self care deficit (requires post void residual bladder scanning and clean intermittent catheterizations), Unilateral
neglect, Impaired skin integrity (Stage 3 pressure ulcer on coccyx)
and Knowledge deficit regarding medical condition. High risk for
falls was identified on admission; she notes that he fell last night
while confused. The Nurse Practitioner (NP) saw him; no injuries
were found, but he is still quite confused this morning. Because he
had an indwelling catheter while hospitalized and is still not empty-
ing his bladder, she is checking for a UTI. The nurse is also wor-
ried because his Coumadin (warfarin) dose is still not stable and
his recent INR was >4. The NP ordered this to be checked STAT
today because of the fall. If he needs an antibiotic, this may affect
his INR further. If his confusion worsens, he will have to go back to
the hospital to be evaluated for a "bleed."*

Discussion

The scenario is abbreviated but you get the idea. On a scale of a good-
better-best ranking in terms of team CT and the "two heads are better
than one" style, how would you rate it?

This typical team meeting in the clinical arena gives everyone some
input, providing opportunities for bringing up problems and concerns,
but that is about the extent of its function. Most team meetings in practice best match the characteristics of a multidisciplinary team, or what
Bensimon and Neumann (1993) would classify as a "Utilitarian Team,"
whose activities consist of "deliver[ing] information, coordinat[ing] and
plan[ning], mak[ing] decisions" (p. 34).

We are sure you came up with a long list to make the team interaction
a better fit with the interdisciplinary column in Table 7.1. For starters,
those changes might include: 1) openly discussing with Mr. D. his desire
to go home and the implications for his safety and that of his wife if he
plans to continue caring for her, 2) discussing options with Mr. D. for
community resources available for his wife's care, and 3) helping Mr. D.

see the patterns of impulsive behavior and implications for his safety. All issues discussed in the meeting are important to patient care, but the team did not move beyond simply sharing information into true collaborative thinking.

Team Thinking in Education

One might assume that nurse educators engage in scholarly team thinking, but, unfortunately, academic nursing educators appear to be even less skilled at interdisciplinary team thinking than nurses in practice. In reality, educators have very little opportunity to collaborate across disciplines. The reward systems in higher education favor independent, not interdependent, thinking.

Here is an opportunity to examine an educator's team meeting and see how thinking occurs.

TACTICS 7.2: Educator Team Meeting and Thinking
1. Read Scenario 7.2 and reflect on the following:
   a. The thinking being demonstrated by the individuals.
   b. The process of thinking as a team.
   c. The outcome of the thinking for achieving one of their goals—increasing nursing student understanding of interdisciplinary team work.
2. Compare this team's characteristics to those in Table 7.1.
3. Make a list of what you would do differently and, to yourself or a colleague, explain why you would do them. Again, use the thinking vocabulary of the 17 dimensions to reflect or share your thinking with a peer.

Scenario 7.2
Educator Team Meeting and Thinking
Janet is the lead nursing faculty in the community health nursing courses. Bob and TaNisha are the other tenured nursing faculty. There are three part-time nursing faculty who teach in the clinical sections of the course. Janet, Bob, and TaNisha each teach a third of the classroom portion of the course. Janet calls a meeting with Bob and TaNisha to review the syllabus for the following year and asks for input.

Bob reminds the others that the paper assignment needs changing; it requires too much grading and he isn't sure students even read all of his extensive feedback on each paper.

TaNisha wants to change the textbook and has a recommendation. TaNisha also shares a need to change how they teach primary, secondary and tertiary prevention, based on the feedback in student evaluations and the low scores on test items in that area.

Janet brings up the need to deal with the new program objective related to increasing students' abilities to work in interdisciplinary teams. She reminds the others of the faculty decision to incorporate that aspect of the IOM recommendations.

Bob suggests a plan to have guest speakers from Occupational Therapy, Physical Therapy and Social Work make presentations to the class and explain their role in patient care.

TaNisha says, "I don't know how we will ever fit that in; we have so much critical information to teach already, I can't give up any of my time. Maybe you or Bob can."

In the end they decide to:

1. *Change the paper assignment to include a peer-reviewed first draft component.*
2. *Change to a newer textbook.*
3. *Add some additional readings on interdisciplinary teamwork to each topic in the course.*

Discussion

What thinking occurred? With regard to individual thinking, we can make a case for *reflection* when Bob and TaNisha looked back at the past year and identified assignments and textbooks that needed modifications. TaNisha also used *logical reasoning* when she drew the inference that, based on low student evaluations of that assignment and low test scores in that content area, a different teaching approach was needed to present primary, secondary and tertiary prevention concepts.

But where is the evidence of team thinking? How did the three think differently as a team than as individuals sharing information? Was team thinking necessary or was this group interaction enough?

This scenario does not even approach the multidisciplinary level of work, let alone IDT thinking, because there are no other disciplines represented. The team in the above scenario consists of only the three educators who teach the classroom content. It does not include the part-time nursing faculty who work with students in the clinical setting to apply classroom concepts. Their viewpoint would have significantly affected the team thinking. Students or even alumni could have added valuable insights as well.

Even with these additional members, however, the thinking would still be limited to nurses. Including faculty from the other disciplines, such as occupational or physical therapy and/or social work, would have increased the probability of an interdisciplinary thinking perspective for both ideas and solutions.

Having examined the terminology of team thinking and looked at some examples of team activities in practice and education, let's now look at who thinks IDTs are important. IDTs have been getting a great deal of support over the last decade because, as Baldwin cited above (1996), they can improve quality healthcare.

Proponents of IDT

The National Academies of Practice convened an expert panel to help guide policy decisions on IDT work (Simpson, et al., 2001). Their goal was to avoid wasting valuable time, money and energy duplicating services, and ensuring that services are not omitted because of assumptions that other providers are doing the care.

The Institute of Medicine (2003) identified the value of IDTs as reducing redundancy of healthcare services and contributing more creative solutions to the complex problems in today's healthcare arena. The Joint Commission on Accreditation of Healthcare Organizations (JCAHO) now requires evidence of interdisciplinary collaboration (Kaissi, Johnson, & Kirschbaum, 2003), and the President's Advisory Committee on Consumer Protection and Quality in the Healthcare Industry recommends all healthcare providers gain more experience in working in interdisciplinary teams (Kaissi, et al., 2003).

In the U.K. the National Health Service has begun what they call the "modernization" agenda. They are expecting not only interdisciplinary, but flexible, teams that cross professional and organizational boundaries. They want to revolutionize healthcare in the U.K. and break down demarcations between different professional groups (Scholes & Vaughan, 2002; Coombs & Dillon, 2002).

These are some pretty influential groups backing IDTs. *Why* do these organizations believe IDTs lead to better patient care? In Baldwin's (1996) review of the literature he found several studies done between the 1960s and early 1990s that reported positive outcomes of IDT work. A summary of the outcomes of those studies indicated that IDTs enhanced patient compliance and satisfaction, reduced costs, decreased hospitalizations, lowered infant and geriatric mortality rates, reduced lengths of stay, and improved staff morale.

A recent large research study by Wheelan, Burchill, & Tilin (2003) examined the impact of IDTs on patient outcomes in 17 ICUs in 9 hospitals in the eastern U.S.A. Two instruments were used—APACHE III to predict risk of dying, and the Group Development Questionnaire to assess staffs' perceptions of their team functioning. At the end of a five-day period, patient mortality was lower on the units where the personnel scored higher on the Group Development Questionnaire. In other words, there was statistically significant evidence to support that units whose staff believed they had effective teamwork in place were units with lower patient mortality rates.

In spite of these positive results we still have need for more research on IDTs. Most IDT literature included recommendations for evidence to clarify how IDTs led to improve patient outcomes (Baldwin, 1996; Fitzpatrick & Montgomery, 2001; Rice, 2000; Simpson, et al., 2001). Studies focusing on the thinking processes in particular would be helpful, as that seems to be assumed or is missing in most IDT literature.

WHAT INTERFERES WITH IDT THINKING?

With all this support for IDT thinking one would expect it to be happening; unfortunately it is not that automatic. We have concluded that four patterns of factors interfere with IDT thinking: personal, professional, communication and timing, and environmental.

Personal Factors

Ego, Ego, Ego. President Harry S. Truman once commented, "It is amazing what you can accomplish if you do not care who gets the credit" ("The Quotations Page" n.d.). If team members need to feel important, believe they have the best ideas, and have difficulty accepting good ideas from other members, team thinking suffers. If team members use the team's thinking time to meet their personal needs for socialization, team thinking suffers.

Mui (2001) described the need for team members to act in concert with each other. If team members have not effectively developed their individual 10 habits of mind and 7 skills in CT, their ability to collaborate, contribute, and act in concert is weakened. For example, if *confidence* in reasoning is not well developed, a person is more easily swayed by the comments of others. If *open-mindedness* is not a strength, biases about a member's or a patient's culture or speech may limit thinking.

Lack of *open-mindedness, flexibility* and *contextual perspective* contribute to low tolerance for ambiguity. If team members are uncomfortable because there are no obvious answers to problems, they are more likely to rush to quick solutions. Quick solutions may ease the anxiety of the team, but they are not always the best solutions. Low tolerance for ambiguity hinders folks from taking the extra time to go beyond acceptable to better or best solutions.

A final personal factor to consider is comfort. How comfortable are you with team membership? For example, what about when patients are present? Will patients' presence prevent you from saying what you really think for fear of hurting their feelings, creating unnecessary worries, or challenging data? How much you value *contextual perspective* may influence your comfort with the patient as a part of the context.

Professional Factors

The first professional factor has to do with discipline autonomy. Nurses have been working very hard since the 1950s to establish their profession as unique, and separate from medicine. They have achieved that goal through the development of a solid knowledge base, research, a code of ethics, and standards of care. However, in the process, they may have also promoted clinicians who avoid collaborative thinking for fear of being traitors to the nursing profession. Nursing, like other disciplines, is a bit ethnocentric—or should we say, discipline-centric? We have been educated in our own domains with our own paradigms for thinking and problem solving. These discipline-autonomy characteristics tend to make us work and think separately, not together. It may be time to apply new professional standards—Interdisciplinary Work Standards, that include strategies for IDT thinking.

The second professional factor interfering with IDT thinking is lack of preparation for team work. Although team work has been given lip service over the last decades, little has been done to achieve it beyond uni-disciplinary teams. For the most part nurses talk with nurses, doctors talk with doctors, nurse educators talk with nurse educators. Because of the nature of their work, social workers, case managers, discharge planners, and community health nurses are probably the groups most skilled at engaging more than one discipline in team thinking and activities. Their jobs require extensive collaboration as they connect clients with necessary resources. Doing that job effectively requires a full understanding of and communication with other disciplines.

In the literature reviewed for this chapter, one message came through loud and clear—the severe lack of interdisciplinary education in all professions (Reeves, 2001; Phillips, et al., 2002; Mac Kinnon & Mac Rae, 1996; Leipzig et al., 2002; IOM, 2003). Limited interdisciplinary education has led to: 1) limited ability to function in practice and education arenas, and 2) underdeveloped professional interaction styles needed to achieve true interdisciplinary collaboration. New models of interdisciplinary education must become a priority in healthcare education in this decade.

The third professional factor influencing CT in teams is leadership. Too much or too little leadership, stifling or encouraging thinking, concern about power and control need to be addressed. According to Simpson et al. (2001) and Siegler (1998), effective IDTs vary leadership depending on the situation at hand. This may be the ideal in theory, but is probably not practical all of the time. However, these variations may stimulate creative configurations.

Communication Factors

The medium of communication and collaborative thinking is language. Discipline-specific language and jargon are cited repeatedly as limiting factors for working in IDTs (Case, 1998; Schofield & Amodeo, 1999). The language of thinking may become the unifying factor for IDT communication and collaboration.

When individuals in the same or different disciplines communicate, conflict is inevitable. One's ability to handle conflict can hinder CT and IDT work. Conflict creates anxiety, which prevents higher order thinking (Hart, 1983). The secret is not to try to eliminate conflict (which, by the way, is impossible), but to use conflict to improve the effectiveness of teams (Sessa, 1998; Northouse & Northouse, 1985). Strategies for improving your ability to use conflict constructively depend on your *confidence* in your reasoning, *flexibility*, and *intellectual integrity*.

An analysis of the current interaction style in healthcare practice and education indicates a developmental delay. Many providers' interaction styles might best be described as parallel play or, at best, multidisciplinary. Parallel play refers to the interaction style used by two- and three-year-old toddlers as they begin their socialization process beyond self. Toddlers using parallel play are aware of others; they enjoy being in the vicinity of others, but basically they do their own thing, not having figured out how to play together. Does this sound like the way we operate sometimes? Moving beyond parallel play to collaborative interactions will likely require *perseverance*.

Timing and Environmental Factors

Time, time management, and lack of time constantly plague healthcare providers. With all the work that needs to be done, it is difficult to convince people that more time needs to be found for meetings within the discipline, let alone interdisciplinary ones. It is even harder to convince folks if their only experience with meetings is wasting time. What's that old saying? A meeting is where you keep minutes but lose hours. Creative solutions for IDT thinking without meetings are proposed later in the chapter. We bet that piqued your interest!

HOW IS THINKING DIFFERENT IN IDT?

The primary solution to the preceding problems is using more than individual CT. We need IDT thinking as well. This section clarifies how CT is different in IDT. With that clarification we can focus on solutions to address the factors that hinder IDT thinking.

The literature on IDT in healthcare seems based on the underlying assumption that CT is a prerequisite for IDT work, but offers little to describe the CT; nor does it demonstrate how team thinking goes beyond individual thinking. To better understand team CT, we must examine literature from other disciplines. Studies of organizations and leadership provided useful guidance for teasing out IDT thinking. Much of that literature is from the business/industry sector, educational leadership and adult learning research.

It is important at this juncture to make a distinction between team thinking and group thinking, or "groupthink." According to Bensimon and Neumann (1993) "groupthink" is a negative term describing what happens when groups mistakenly assume harmony is the way to achieve group goals. Originating in the early 1970s, "groupthink" described a phenomenon of "assumed consensus" that discouraged group members from voicing their concerns, doubts, points of view, or sharing data that did not fit with the predominant conclusions. Groupthink does not describe CT; groupthink describes a quick method to reach a conclusion, a very different phenomenon.

If "groupthink" is the antithesis of CT, where does that leave us? Are there ways for team members to pool their thinking without settling for "groupthink"? The answer is yes, and one solution is "systems thinking." Senge (1990) explained how to use systems thinking to create team-oriented learning organizations in business. As shown in Box 7.1 on page 130, systems thinking goes beyond the thinking of the individual and helps counter some of the linear thinking adults have been molded into over the years. Systems thinking is ideally suited for IDT work.

Senge believed the key to systems thinking was dialogue among members of the team as they "enter into a genuine 'thinking together'" (p. 10). Genuine thinking together requires that thinkers suspend assumptions and allow for "free flowing of meaning through the group, allowing the group to discover insights not attainable individually" (p. 10). At the IOM Summit (2003) the language of system-mindedness was used to capture this same idea—cooperation and thinking together.

Ubbes, Black, and Ausherman (1999) believed systems thinking was a tool for thinkers to modify their "value dualisms" of linear thinking (yes/no, black/white, body/mind) to their more real world dimensions of yes/no/maybe, black/white/gray, mind/body/spirit. They described systems thinking as the

---

Box 7.1

Senge's (1990) View: Systems Thinking is . . .

- A discipline of seeing wholes, seeing inter-relationships rather than things, seeing patterns of change vs. static snapshots.
- Recognizing that members are part of that pattern, not separate from the patterns.
- Seeing relationships vs. linear cause and effect chains of actions.
- The ability to avoid merely shifting problems around, making today's solutions tomorrow's problems.
- Recognizing that our basic skills in systems thinking are underdeveloped or repressed by formal education in linear thinking. Reality is made up of circles, but we tend to see only straight lines that limit our systems thinking.
- A process that requires more dialogue than discussion, interactions of the mind as opposed to simply sharing information.

---

means to see multiple perspectives and broaden understanding by recognizing relationships between and among pieces of data.

Bensimon and Neumann (1993) have used the term "team thinking" in their writings about collective thinking. Figure 7.2, based on their findings, is an illustration of the continuum of team types and the different thinking at the ends of that continuum. The ideal is on the far right and may not be realistic for all organizations in healthcare or education, but it gives us a direction to strive for. Remember, in reality, clinicians and educators often need to adapt ideas and create hybrid teams to work in their worlds. Use this illustration to visualize some of the gradations of IDT thinking before reading about them in more detail.

Bensimon and Neumann (1993) conducted a comprehensive qualitative research study to identify the thinking necessary for teams to function effectively in higher education settings. They studied leadership teams in 15 universities in the U.S.A. over a three-year period, making two visits to each university over that period of time. They identified several patterns of thinking skills necessary for effective team functioning and described "thinking as a conglomerate verb, referring to a wide variety of mental processes (for example, defining, analyzing, synthesizing)" (p. 59).

Bensimon and Neumann used the terminology of "team thinking" to represent "The Art of Thinking Together,"(p. 55), a condition necessary to move from "utilitarian" style teams to "cognitive" style teams. Utilitarian style teams sim-

Figure 7.2 Continuum of Thinking in Teams

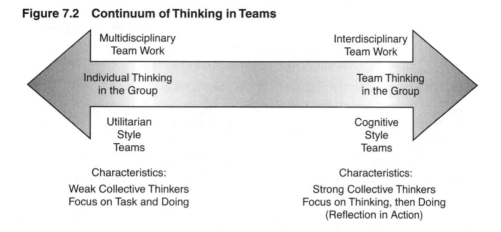

Multidisciplinary Team Work	Interdisciplinary Team Work
Individual Thinking in the Group	Team Thinking in the Group
Utilitarian Style Teams	Cognitive Style Teams

Characteristics:

Weak Collective Thinkers
Focus on Task and Doing

Characteristics:

Strong Collective Thinkers
Focus on Thinking, then Doing
(Reflection in Action)

ply achieve tasks and their members are generally weak at collective thinking. Cognitive style thinking teams, or real teams, achieve more than task completion. These authors believed that doing a task was only the tip of the iceberg of real team work. The inner workings of real teams, not visible in task outcomes, includes "team members' thinking, talking, wondering, asking, speculating, arguing, correcting, trying, rethinking, creating, trying again" (p. 55).

According to Bensimon and Neumann, real teams functioning at the cognitive level recognize their purpose as "sense making." In real teams,

> . . . its members are collectively involved in perceiving, analyzing, learning, and thinking . . . the team is a brainlike social structure that enlarges the intelligence span of individual team members . . . allows the group to behave as a creative system . . . a) viewing problems from multiple perspectives, b) questioning, challenging, and arguing, and c) acting as a monitor and feedback system (p. 41).

From their research, Bensimon and Neumann (1993) identified eight member thinking roles when teams functioned effectively—five core roles of team thinking and three support thinking roles. Any of the eight roles can be assumed by different individuals over time and/or can change during the course of the discussions, but, the more thinking roles that are present, the better the team thinks. Box 7.2 includes their eight roles with brief descriptions. Attention to these roles helps team members become aware of group thinking processes, what is helping and what is hindering achievement of IDT goals.

Brookfield and Preskill (1999) offered another perspective on team thinking. They referred to " 'group talk' as a blending of conversation, discussion and dialogue . . . to create new meanings, [incorporating] reciprocity . . . , exchange and inquiry, cooperation and collaboration . . . " (p. 6). They went on

Box 7.2

Eight Team Thinking Roles identified by Bensimon and Neumann (1993).

1. The definer (voices and creates the team's reality)
2. The analyst (assesses all the parts of the issue)
3. The interpreter (provides insight on how outcomes might be perceived)
4. The critic (re-defines and re-analyzes and re-interprets)
5. The synthesizer (elicits all thinking perspectives and helps provide linkages for solutions)
6. The disparity monitor (assesses how outcomes are perceived)
7. The task monitor (removes obstacles to team thinking and facilitates the team work)
8. The emotional monitor (addresses the human, personal and emotional aspects of team thinking during the thinking process)

to describe thinking habits of collaboration that include critical analysis and reflective speculation.

Brookfield and Preskill made a strong case for how discussion enhances learning through the cultivation of critical reflection and thinking. They offered strategies promoting CT through discussion with exercises called "Critical Incident Questionnaires" (p. 49), "Telling Tales from the Trenches" (p. 77), and "Circle of Voices" (p. 80), to name just a few.

Bensimon and Neumann (1993) and Brookfield and Preskill (1999) recommended group self assessment and reflection to monitor thinking and its outcomes. We have created a Team Thinking Inventory (Box 7.3) based on their ideas as well as Senge's to help clinicians and educators do both pre and post assessment of their team thinking. You now have an opportunity to try it yourself.

TACTICS 7.3: Team Thinking Assessment

This activity can be performed by both clinicians and educators.

1. Select a team of which you are a member.
2. Think about the function of that team, its purpose, the way it operates and the ways in which its members participate. Compare the

functioning to Figure 7.2 and see where on the Utilitarian–Cognitive Continuum your team fits.

3. Using the Team Thinking Inventory (Box 7.3), assess that team.
4. Compare the behaviors demonstrated by team members with the Eight Team Thinking Roles in Box 7.2

Box 7.3

Team Thinking Inventory
(adapted from Senge, 1990, Bensimon & Neumann, 1993, and Brookfield & Preskill, 1999)

1. What strategies are used to help team members think about the big picture as well as the parts?
2. What strategies are used to help team members see the situation from different perspectives?
3. What strategies are used to help team members see their biases and assumptions?
4. What strategies help team members think about patterns and inter-relationships of issues and parts of problems?
5. What strategies are used to help team members think beyond cause and effect consequences?
6. Does the thinking that occurs in the team resemble simple sharing of information or discussion/dialogue? Why? How can you move in the direction of discussion/dialogue?
7. What is done to encourage team members to share their thinking or feel comfortable enough to talk about it?
8. How is conflict managed in the team to promote thinking instead of discouraging it?
9. What other sources of gratification are available for team members to socialize, obtain recognition and interact, besides interdisciplinary team work?
10. How were the interdisciplinary team members prepared for their thinking roles?
11. How does the team deal with ambiguity? How long can they tolerate not having a solution?
12. How does the team examine its own thinking processes, e.g. *how* it works, not *what* it is doing and *who* is doing it?

Discussion

What did you discover? Does your team function at the Utilitarian or the Cognitive end of the continuum or somewhere in between? How did the team thinking manifest itself on the Team Thinking Inventory? Which of the eight thinking roles were present and which were not? What can you and the others on the team do to modify your team thinking? These are tough questions and the answers probably require more than your CT. It may be time to share this activity with the team and get some team thinking going.

Now let's eavesdrop on another team meeting in healthcare that demonstrates some team/systems thinking. Scenario 7.3 represents an in-patient psychiatric unit interdisciplinary team meeting.

TACTICS 7.4: Finding the IDT Thinking

Read the somewhat condensed dialogue of Scenario 7.3. Identify aspects that do or do not fit with team /systems thinking.

Scenario 7.3

Intake Note:

Mary James is a 34-year-old Caucasian married female with two children ages 3 and 1. She was admitted yesterday in the early afternoon to the inpatient psychiatric unit with suicidal ideation and the following DSM-IV-TR Axis I diagnosis was made: Major depressive disorder: recurrent with generalized weakness.

Psychiatric History: *One episode of Post-Partum Depression after second child born. Wellbutrin was effective after trying several different antidepressants but was discontinued by the patient after 6 months.* ***Intake Nursing Assessment:*** *Pt has lost 10# over the last three months, little appetite. Denies ETOH intake, denies smoking, drinks about 8–10 cups of coffee a day. Complains of problems sleeping, averaging 2–3 hours per night for the last three months. Very tired and having difficulty keeping up with child-care; husband has had to take off work to help out during the day. Husband appears very supportive but concerned about the re-occurrence of depression. All other assessment data WNL.*

Beginning dialogue occurring during the first interdisciplinary team meeting after Mrs. James' admission

Social worker: *"Mr. James, we are meeting as a team to plan for your wife's care and encourage you to be an active participant until your wife is able to join us. Welcome to the team."*

Mr. James: "Thanks. I don't know what I can do, but I'll do what I can."

Nurse: "We include patients and/or family members on the team to help make sure we don't miss important pieces of information unique to their situation. It makes for safer, quicker, and better care. We also want you to help with making decisions."

Psychiatrist: "I assume we have all read Mrs. James' history. According to Mr. James and his wife, they believe this recent episode of depression and suicidal ideation began building after Joy, their second child, was born. Outpatient treatment and re-starting bupropion have not been successful. I'm thinking we need to try one of the newer SSRIs. I want to wean her off bupropion for a couple of days and then try escitalopram to see if we can't attack different neurotransmitters sites."

Physical therapist: "Mr. James, did you understand all that?"

Mr. James: "Not exactly."

Psychiatrist: "Sorry about that. Let me translate that doctor jargon. Your wife is experiencing a clinical depression. All of the symptoms you described about her not eating, having trouble sleeping, thinking about hurting herself, etc. all fit with that diagnosis. Basically the chemicals in her brain that affect how she feels are not working properly and that brings on these symptoms. These chemical imbalances can be triggered by pregnancy and childbirth. The medication your wife was taking, Wellbutrin, is one way to treat depression. When one way doesn't work, we need to try something else. Luckily, there are several to choose from, and I would like to try one called Lexapro. It is in a different classification of antidepressants meaning it works on different parts of the brain and therefore may work better. Does that help?"

Mr. James: "Yes."

Physical therapist: "I've done a preliminary eval. and think we can start some strengthening activities slowly. Mrs. James has really lost a lot of muscle mass; besides the activity will stimulate some endorphins and help with the depression as well."

Mr. James: "But what about her headache? It was getting worse all yesterday and no better when I had to leave at 4:00 to get the kids from the neighbors." (Starts to get tears in his eyes.) "I'm afraid she might have a brain tumor because the medicine you ordered yesterday didn't help at all."

Psychiatrist: "Let's not jump to conclusions about tumors, but what's going on with the headache?" (looking to the nurse)

Nurse: *"I think we figured out what the headaches are about. Last night the student nurse working with your wife did an excellent assessment and we realized that her caffeine intake has significantly changed since admission. Since there was no reason to restrict caffeine we made sure she had a couple cups of coffee before and during dinner. She told the night nurse the headache was almost gone."*

Mr. James: *"She does drink lots of coffee. She says it helps her get through the day."*

Psychiatrist: *"Caffeine shouldn't be a problem; she can have her coffee, so lets move on to the depression issues."*

Nutritionist: *"Before we skip over caffeine and nutrition too quickly, let's talk about how it can contribute to the depression. I haven't had an opportunity to meet with Mrs. James yet, but, from what I've heard it sounds like her nutritional intake or lack of nutrients along with lack of activity"* (looking at physical therapist) *"might be contributing as well. I would also like to share some of the new research on Omega 3 Fatty Acids and treating depression. . . . "*

Social Worker: *"I think we should also explore Mr. James' comment about a brain tumor to see what is behind that concern and then, Dr. Jones, could you explain to him what you would do to rule out that possibility?"*

This dialogue continued focusing on treating the depression and the suicidal ideation, ongoing contracting for safety, combinations of medication, activity and nutritional changes, exploring existing and new ways of coping for the family, including resources to help Mr. James with child care during is wife's hospitalization and support groups for the parents after discharge. Each professional then shared what specifically he or she would focus on for discharge planning as well as the day's care.

Discussion

Wasn't finding the group thinking a very challenging task? It is really hard to clearly identify actual thinking by an individual or a group. You probably used some of the same comparisons you chose for TACTICS 7.3 to help find the thinking. Although the thinking in this team was moving in the right direction and there was somewhat more discussion, it still has a long way to go to achieve true interdisciplinary collaboration.

An Example of an Effective IDT

Effective teams in healthcare are increasing. One example is PACE (Program for All-Inclusive Care for the Elderly), a team model for managed long-term care (Mui, 2001). This model was designed to provide the frail elderly with options for living in communities instead of nursing homes. The goals of the program were to maximize the residents' autonomy while providing quality at lower costs.

Based on a British day hospital concept, the first PACE program was developed in San Francisco in 1971. As of 2001 there were 70 organizations in 30 states operating at different stages of the PACE model, serving over 9,000 frail elderly. Their interdisciplinary team members include social workers, nurses, physicians, physical therapists, occupational therapists, recreational therapists, home health aides, pharmacists, psychologists, psychiatrists, dentists, durable medical equipment suppliers, hospice staff, housing personnel and chaplains.

It has taken over 25 years to move from conception to supportive legislation and nationwide implementation of the PACE model, but it is working. A key factor making it successful was identified as the team that is "competent and strong in their individual disciplines and have the skills and attitudes to work collaboratively to achieve broader objectives . . . " (Mui, 2001, p. 64). Mui cited the team members' courage to embrace change from traditional forms of care to this collaborative approach.

CULTIVATING IDT THINKING FOR CLINICIANS AND EDUCATORS

Thinking in an effective team environment does not happen automatically; it takes time, effort, and a commitment to think beyond your discipline's knowledge bases, aspirations and values (McCormack, 2001; Salmon & Jones, 2001). It also takes a shift in organizational culture to mutually respect working partnerships (Coombs, 2001). Bottom line: cultivating IDT thinking is hard work. We do not have any magic bullets, but we have some helpful suggestions.

For starters, not all IDT thinking requires meetings. The IOM talks about IDT *work*, not IDT meetings. This is an important distinction and helps us to think outside that ol' box! This awareness can lead to all kinds of *creativity* and *flexibility* to change the IDT *work* environment mind-set for clinicians and educators.

Clinicians

The IOM (2003) summarized eight conditions necessary for effective IDT work in the practice setting. Although they do not overtly mention thinking, we believe if you examine Box 7.4, you will decide it is impossible to achieve anything on the list without thinking. These too can all occur in providers' daily interactions in addition to meetings.

Case (1998) identified several similar factors that need to be in place for teamwork to occur in the practice setting: 1) a common language, 2) a common

---

Box 7.4

IOM conditions for effective IDT work (IOM, 2003, p. 56)

- Learn about other team members' expertise, background, knowledge, and values.
- Learn individual roles and processes required to work collaboratively.
- Demonstrate basic group skills, including communication, negotiation, delegation, time management, and assessment of group dynamics.
- Ensure that accurate and timely information reaches those who need it at the appropriate times.
- Customize care and manage smooth transitions across settings and over time, even when the team members are in entirely different physical locations.
- Coordinate and integrate care processes to ensure excellence, continuity, and reliability of the care provided.
- Resolve conflicts with other members of the team.
- Communicate with other members of the team in a shared language, even when the members are in entirely different physical locations.

---

knowledge base, 3) shared core values, 4) understanding the roles of the team members, 5) respect for team members, and 6) mutual sharing among the members. Case encouraged staff development specialists to pay attention to these factors when they promote IDT *work*. Note that Case did not say "meetings." All of her recommendations can occur in corridor discussions as long as privacy issues are maintained of course.

An excellent example of non-meeting IDT thinking is offered by Halm, Goering and Smith (2003) with the use of Interdisciplinary Rounds (IDR). IDT are enhanced discharge planning rounds in which each discipline reviews the patient record, identifies problems from the discipline's perspective, shares information with the team, collaborates on approaches, identifies barriers to the approaches, and identifies individual and team learning needs. The goals for IDR were timely and safe discharges, improved documentation of collaborative care, and increased awareness of each disciplines skills and resources.

They implemented IDR in a large midwestern hospital on medicine, orthopedics, neurology, rehabilitation, surgery, cardiology, oncology, behavioral health and the birthing center units. The plan was to use IDR as a means of engaging all disciplines in discharge planning. Participating clinical nurse specialists used the Internet to collaborate with other institutions using similar processes. Sharing of ideas and constant modifications took place as new information became available. At the end of six months outcomes of the IDR included: "greater participation by all the disciplines in achieving patient and family outcomes, increased early recognition of patients at risk, and improved communication among member of the healthcare team" (p. 133).

Educators

The IOM conditions for effective IDT in Box 7.4 are also valuable in the educational setting. Their implementation will be a challenge because IDT activities are not generally rewarded. Value in education has traditionally been given to independent work. These traditions must be changed to prepare educators and students of all the professions for IDT practice in the real world.

Rice (2000) recommended a dual socialization process in academic education. For example, nursing students would not only learn their profession, but would have courses and clinical experiences together with students from other disciplines; as a result of thinking and working together as groups they would learn to share and respect each other from the start. Rice based her recommendation on her experience as a social worker and her extensive literature review of 302 articles.

Some professional education programs are taking IDT concepts to heart. Two deans in Colorado, one from a medical school and one from a nursing school, worked together to change scheduling so that students in those programs could take courses together (personnel communication, Peter Pronovost, MD, PhD, March 28, 2004).

We have firsthand knowledge of one IDT course that has been very successful. Faculty from the Schools of Nursing, Social Work and the School of Associated Health Professions at Eastern Michigan University worked collaboratively to develop and teach a course called "Aging to Infancy: A Retrospective Approach to Life." The disciplines involved were nursing, social work, occupational therapy and dietetics. All four faculty participated before, during and after the class periods to coordinate their teaching, discuss issues arising in class, and assess students' learning. A major goal of this course was to demonstrate to students how the disciplines collaborate in both thinking and doing to address healthcare issues across age groups. Course enrollment increased from 25 students the first year to over 100 two years later.

Educational collaboration across disciplines is also being encouraged at policy making levels. For example, a suggestion was made at the American Association of Colleges of Nursing (AACN) pre-meeting in March of 2004 to invite deans of medical schools and other disciplines to future AACN annual meetings to identify curricular challenges and opportunities for more interdisciplinary teaching. Recommendations from AACN may ultimately be translated into accreditation requirements by the Commission on Collegiate Nursing Education (CCNE), and those requirements drive curricular changes.

Before making too many curricular changes, however, we need new models for teaching IDT. More research is necessary to develop those IDT models (Reeves, 2001; Scholes & Vaughan, 2002). Those models must include overt thinking processes and structured academic experiences to prepare students before they enter the workforce (Mac Kinnon & Mac Rae, 1996; Leipzig, et al., 2002). And in the meantime, educators from different disciplines can make conscious efforts to talk to each other, explore portions of course work that can be done collaboratively, and create opportunities for students to value IDT thinking and IDT work. These pilot projects will lead to models for research in professional curricula.

Whether in practice or education, initial efforts to enhance IDT work will take time, energy and thinking. It may seem overwhelming; you will want to fall back on, "It's easier to do it myself." At first we will likely continue using hybrid versions of IDT. But once IDT thinking is integrated into daily activities that go beyond having more meetings, the time factor becomes less of an issue.

PAUSE AND PONDER:
FUTURE IMPLICATION OF IDT THINKING

Moving toward IDT thinking is no longer a choice; it is a necessity. We must value IDT and develop leaders in practice and education who promote, cultivate, and nurture IDT thinking. Today's clinicians may have to learn IDT thinking on the job, but hopefully tomorrow's will have learned IDT thinking in school.

Reflection Cues

- Interdisciplinary teams (IDTs) are essential for dealing with the increasing complexity of healthcare.
- Most team meetings in practice best match the characteristics of a multidisciplinary team or a "Utilitarian Team" whose activities consist of delivering information, coordinating and planning, and making decisions.
- IDTs focus on collaborative problem identification as well as problem solving.
- IDTs occur less frequently in academic settings than in practice settings.
- Research studies indicate that IDTs: enhances patient compliance, produces greater patient satisfaction, reduces costs, decreases in hospital-

izations, lowers infant and geriatric mortality rates, reduces lengths of stay and improves staff morale.

- Personal, professional, communication, time and environmental factors can interfere with team thinking.

- Discipline autonomy tends to promote working and thinking separately and not together.

- Lack of preparation and training to work in IDTs is a major impediment to IDT work.

- Thinking in IDTs is more than simply adding ideas together; IDT thinking blends ideas and creates new ones that individuals would not have considered independently.

- Attention to Bensimon and Neumann's (1993) eight thinking roles of teams is helpful in assessing IDT work.

- Not all IDT thinking requires meetings; Interdisciplinary Rounds are one alternative.

- Educational models and research are needed to demonstrate effective IDT strategies and outcomes.

- IDT work takes time and energy, effective leadership and critical thinking to be successful.

References

Baldwin Jr., D. C. (1996). Some historical notes on interdisciplinary and interprofessional education and practice in healthcare in the USA. *Journal of Interprofessional Care, 10* (2), 173–187.

Bensimon, E. M. & Neumann, A. (1993). *Redesigning collegiate leadership: Teams and teamwork in higher education.* Baltimore: The Johns Hopkins University Press.

Brookfield, S. D. & Preskill, S. (1999). *Discussion as a way of teaching: Tools and techniques for Democratic classrooms.* San Francisco: Jossey-Bass.

Case, B. (1998). Competency development: Critical thinking, clinical judgment, and technical ability. In Karen J. Kelly-Thomas (Ed.) *Clinical and nursing staff development: Current competency, future focus.* 2nd Ed., (pp. 240–281). Philadelphia: Lippincott.

Coombs, M. (2001). Towards collaborative and collegial caring: A comparative study. *Nursing in Critical Care, 6* (1), 23–27.

Coombs, M. & Dillon, A. (2002). Crossing boundaries, re-defining care: The role of the critical care outreach team. *Journal of Clinical Nursing, 11,* 387–397.

Fitzpatrick, J. J. & Montgomery, K. S. (2001). Investment in the future: Interdisciplinary education for primary care. *Issues in Interdisciplinary Care, 3* (1), 77–81.

Halm, M. A., Goering, M. & Smith, M. (2003). Interdisciplinary rounds: Impact on patients, families, and staff. *Clinical Nurse Specialist, 17* (3), 133–142.

Hart, L. A. (1983). *Human brain and human learning.* New York: Longman.

Institute of Medicine (2003). *Health professions education: A bridge to quality.* Washington, DC: The National Academies Press.

Kaissi, A., Johnson, T, & Kirschbaum, M. S. (2003). Measuring teamwork and patient safety attitudes of high-risk areas. *Nursing Economics, 21* (5), 211–218.

Leipzig, R. M., Hyer, K., Ek, K., Wallenstein, S., Vezina, M.L., Fairchild, S., Cassel, C.K., & Howe, J. L. (2002). Attitudes toward working on interdisciplinary healthcare teams: A comparison by discipline. *Journal of the American Geriatrics Society, 50* (6), 1141–1148.

Mac Kinnon, J. L. & Mac Rae, N. (1996). Fostering geriatric interdisciplinary collaboration through academic education. *Physical & Occupational Therapy in Geriatrics, 14* (3), 41–49.

McCormack, B. (2001). Clinical effectiveness and clinical teams: Effective practice with older people. *Nursing Older People, 13* (5), 14–17.

Mui, A. C. (2001). The Program of All-Inclusive Care for the Elderly (PACE): An innovative long-term care model in the United States. *Journal of Aging & Social Policy, 13* (2/3), 53–67.

Northouse, P. G. & Northouse, L. L. (1985). *Health communication: A handbook for health professionals.* Englewood Cliffs, NJ: Prentice-Hall.

Phillips, R. L., Harper, D. C., Wakefield, M., Green, L. A., & Fryer Jr., G. E. (2002). Can nurse practitioners and physicians beat parochialism into plowshares? *Health Affairs, 21* (5), 133–139.

Reeves, S. (2001). A systematic review of the effects of interprofessional education on staff involved in the care of adults with mental health problems. *Journal of Psychiatric and Mental Health Nursing, 8,* 533–542.

Rice, A. H. (2000). Interdisciplinary collaboration in healthcare: Education, practice and research. *National Academies of Practice Forum, 2* (1), 59–73.

Salmon, D. & Jones, M. (2001). Shaping the interprofessional agenda: A study examining qualified nurses' perceptions of learning with others. *Nurse Education Today, 21,* 18–25.

Schofield, R. F. & Amodeo, M. (1999). Interdisciplinary teams in healthcare and human service settings: Are they effective? *Health and Social Work, 24* (3), 210–219.

Scholes, J. & Vaughan, B. (2002). Cross boundary working: Implications for the multiprofessional team. *Journal of Clinical Nursing, 11,* 399–408.

Senge, P. M. (1990). *The fifth discipline: The art and practice of the learning organization.* New York: Doubleday.

Sessa, V. (1998). Professional development initiative: Using conflict to improve effectiveness of nurse teams. *Orthopaedic Nursing, 17* (3), 41–46.

Siegler, E. L. (1998). *Geriatric interdisciplinary team training.* New York: Springer.

Simpson, G., Rabin, D., Schmitt, M., Taylor, P., Urban, S., & Ball, J. (2001). Interprofessional healthcare practice: Recommendations of the National Academies of Practice expert panel on healthcare in the 21st century. *Issues in Interdisciplinary Care, 3* (1), 5–19.

The quotations page (n.d.). Retrieved August 11, 2004, from http://www.quotationspage.com/quotes.php3?author+Harry+S+Truman

Ubbes, V. A., Black, J. M. & Ausherman, J. A. (1999). Teaching for understanding in health education: The role of critical and creative thinking skills within constructivism theory. *Journal of Health Education, 30,* (2), 67–72.

Wheelan, S. A., Burchill, C. N., & Tilin, F. (2003). The link between teamwork and patients' outcomes in intensive care units. *American Journal of Critical Care, 12* (6), 527–534.

CHAPTER 8

Critical Thinking and Evidence-Based Practice

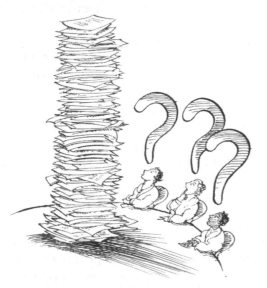

"ALL THIS RESEARCH AND WE STILL HAVE QUESTIONS."

Evidence-based practice (EBP) and its various synonymous cousins (e.g., evidence-based medicine and evidence-based nursing) reveal a very important paradigm shift in how healthcare is practiced and taught. There are many definitions of EBP, as seen in Box 8.1. One thing they all have in common is a move away from basing practice merely on tradition—doing things the way they've always been done without questioning whether that is the best approach—and moving toward basing practice decisions on the best available knowledge (evidence). The Institute of Medicine (2003) envisioned EBP as "the integration of best research evidence, clinical expertise, and patient values in making decisions about the care of individual patients" (p. 56). They clarified "best research evidence" as quantitative evidence such as clinical

Box 8.1

Definitions of Evidence-Based Practice

The IOM (2003): EBP is "the integration of best research evidence, clinical expertise, and patient values in making decisions about the care of individual patients" (p. 56).

Sackett, Richardson, Rosenberg, and Haynes (1997): "Evidence-based medicine . . . is the conscientious explicit and judicious use of current best evidence in making decisions about the care of individual patient. The practice of evidence-based medicine means integrating individual clinical expertise with the best available external clinical evidence from systematic research" (p. 2).

Evidence-Based Clinical Practice Working Group (n.d.): "Clinicians who wish to practice evidence-based health care require the following skills:
• Defining clinical questions in a way that allows clear answers
• Efficient searching for the best information to answer the question
• Appraising the evidence to determine its strength
• Extracting the clinical message from the information
• Applying that information to ones' patients" (para 2).

Driever (2002): "Evidence on which nursing practice is based is derived from the synthesis of knowledge from research; data analyzed from the medical record; quality improvement and risk data; infection control data; international, national and local standards; pathophysiology; cost effectiveness analysis; benchmarking data; patient preferences; and clinical expertise. Evidence-based Nursing Practice involves the explicit and judicious decision making about health care delivery for individuals or groups of patients based on the consensus of the most relevant and supported evidence derived from theory-derived research and data-based information to respond to consumers' preferences and societal expectations" (p. 589).

Stetler, et al., 1998): "Evidence-based nursing deemphasizes ritual, isolated and unsystematic clinical experiences, ungrounded opinions and tradition as a basis for nursing practices . . . and stresses instead the use of research findings and, as appropriate, quality improvement data, other operational and evaluation data, the consensus of recognized experts and affirmed experience to substantiate practice" (p. 48–49).

trials and laboratory experiments, evidence from qualitative research, and evidence from experts in practice. "Clinical expertise" comes from knowledge and experience over time. "Patient values" are those unique circumstances of each patient.

The IOM (2003) enumerated several tasks necessary to EBP: 1) knowing where and how to find best evidence, 2) formulating clinical questions, 3) searching for answers to those questions with the best evidence and determining the validity and appropriateness of that evidence for patient populations, and 4) determining how and when to integrate those new findings in practice. As you can already see, each of these tasks is primarily a thinking process.

Increasingly we are seeing links between thinking and EBP in the literature; even when the links aren't explicit, there is an implication that the very nature of EBP necessitates critical thinking. Profetto-McGrath, Hesketh, Lang, and Estabrooks (2003) found a significant correlation between critical thinking dispositions and research utilization, which is a precursor and close relative of EBP. Higgs, Burn, and Jones (2001) argued that, with the uncertainty of clinical practice contexts, evidence-based practice must be integrated with clinical reasoning. Youngblut and Brooten (2001) focused on the critical thinking in this observation: "Evidence-based practice demands that clinicians look critically at the foundation of their practice and identify which practices are based on research evidence, which are based on clinical knowledge and which are based on tradition" (p. 473). Stetler's group came right out and said, "Inherent to EBP are critical thinking and research utilization competencies" (Stetler et al., 1998, p. 49). Sams and Gannon (2000) also were blunt in stating that EBP ". . . demands critical thinking . . ." (p. 126).

With EBP, one must decide when it is necessary to search for evidence (delineating clinical questions), what constitutes evidence, where and how it can be found, the quality of that evidence, how best to translate that evidence into practice, the potential consequences of using approaches advocated by the evidence, and, after using it, how to determine if it was "best" (Centre for Health Evidence, 2001; "Evidence-based clinical . . ." n.d.). That statement alone implies use of the CT skills of *analyzing, applying standards, discriminating, information seeking, logical reasoning, predicting,* and *transforming knowledge.* It also implies habits of the mind such as *contextual perspective, inquisitiveness, intellectual integrity,* and *open-mindedness.*

Indeed, a clear connection between all dimensions of CT and EBP can be made. Figure 8.1 illustrates the interrelationships as the various CT skills and habits of the mind are superimposed on the components of EBP. Because CT skills and habits of the mind are used in harmony, there is no absolute step in the EBP process where only one or two CT dimensions are used alone. However, certain parts of the EBP process demand more of some skills and habits of the mind than do others. We will return to this figure and more discussion of the thinking pieces after we look at the history of EBP. The history of this movement is very helpful for understanding its importance and how closely aligned with CT it has been since its inception.

Figure 8.1   Inter-relationships of CT Skills and Habits of the Mind and Components of EBP

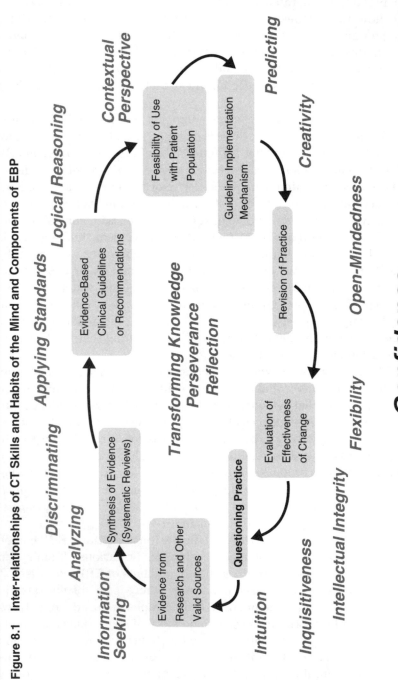

HISTORICAL OVERVIEW OF EBP

While Sackett, Richardson, Rosenberg, and Haynes (1997) attributed the historical roots of EBP to 19th century Paris or earlier, most people give credit to Archie Cochrane, a British physician who, in the 1970s, saw a need to examine the economics of healthcare and determine the cost/benefit of treatments. In 1993 Cochrane and others founded the Cochrane Collaboration that has become the core of EBP ("The name behind . . .," 2004). The Cochrane Collaboration focuses on interventions, precise and thorough searches and evaluation of evidence, and considers the randomized controlled trial (RCT) as the gold standard of research evidence (Jennings & Loan, 2001).

Coining the term *Evidence-Based Medicine* in the 1980s, on this side of the ocean, Canadians at McMaster Medical School in Hamilton, Ontario, are generally credited with making this new critical approach to medical education and practice a reality (Sackett et al., (1997). The Evidence Based Medicine Working Group (EBMWG), now called the Evidence-Based Clinical Practice Working Group (EBCP), formed there and continues to be a leader in this important movement ("Evidence-based clinical . . .," n.d.). The McMaster approach heralded a move away from valuing authority to valuing research as a basis of learning.

Meanwhile, in the United States, the Federal Government committed money in the early 1990s to set up the Agency for Health Care Policy and Reform (AHCPR) that established interdisciplinary teams to gather and assess available literature and develop evidence-based clinical guidelines. Those early guidelines addressed very important areas of health care. Examples of early guidelines were *Pressure Ulcer Treatment, Depression in Primary Care,* and *Management of Cancer Pain.* For those of us who grabbed these guidelines as if they were gold, we soon realized that we had reached a new era of practice— when it wasn't just up to us to keep up with the latest research; someone else valued our desire to provide the best care using the best evidence. Nurses were prominent members of the interdisciplinary teams who did this early work. AHCPR was changed to the Agency for Healthcare Research and Quality (AHRQ) in the mid 1990s (http://www.ahrq.gov) and now has a clearinghouse for clinical guidelines (http://www.guidelines.gov) and has established 12 EBP Centers in the USA (AHRQ, 2002; Evidence-based Practice Centers, n.d.).

Other aspects of nursing history are also very important to the EBP movement. In the late 1970s and early 1980s nursing groups on both sides of this country started focusing on research utilization. Of particular note is the Conduct and Utilization of Research in Nursing (CURN) project in Michigan. Seventeen hospitals in Michigan participated in developing research-based protocols in pre- and post-operative teaching, reducing diarrhea in tube fed

patients, and several other areas (Haller, Reynolds & Horsley, 1979). Unfortunately, although this group and its many followers pushed for increased use of
research in nursing, there continued to be a gap between research and practice in the field. However, the research utilization movement provided fertile
ground for nursing to wholeheartedly embrace the EBP movement.

By 1998 the *Evidence-Based Nursing Journal* was started by a Canadian
and British group. In Australia, The Joanna Briggs Institute (JBI) has become a
model of nursing focused EBP, conducting systematic reviews and developing
evidence-based clinical guidelines and maintaining an excellent website used
by nurses all over the world (http://www.joannabriggs.edu.au).

Today, one can find vast amounts of material on the Internet relative to
EBP. In Chapter 9, "Informatics," we discuss this subject more fully. For the
current chapter we have compiled in Box 8.2 a few of our favorite sites. If you
look at these sites you can find links to hundreds more. Because the EBP and
Informatics movements are growing so rapidly, by the time you read this book
there will likely be many other sites to be found. A general search with the
words "evidence-based practice" will give you lots of strong hits. You need
very little information-seeking ability to find EBP resources.

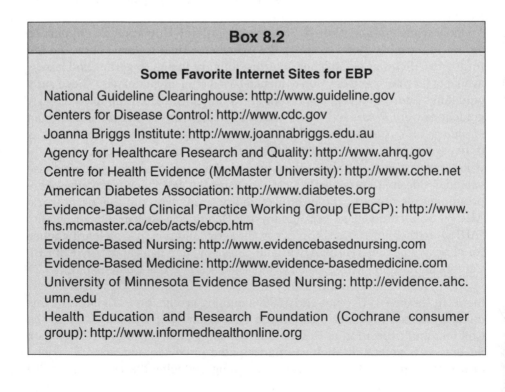

Box 8.2

Some Favorite Internet Sites for EBP

National Guideline Clearinghouse: http://www.guideline.gov

Centers for Disease Control: http://www.cdc.gov

Joanna Briggs Institute: http://www.joannabriggs.edu.au

Agency for Healthcare Research and Quality: http://www.ahrq.gov

Centre for Health Evidence (McMaster University): http://www.cche.net

American Diabetes Association: http://www.diabetes.org

Evidence-Based Clinical Practice Working Group (EBCP): http://www.
fhs.mcmaster.ca/ceb/acts/ebcp.htm

Evidence-Based Nursing: http://www.evidencebasednursing.com

Evidence-Based Medicine: http://www.evidence-basedmedicine.com

University of Minnesota Evidence Based Nursing: http://evidence.ahc.
umn.edu

Health Education and Research Foundation (Cochrane consumer
group): http://www.informedhealthonline.org

A significant new phase of EBP's history is happening right now: the Cochrane group has started addressing the need to include health consumers in its audience (White, 2002). The Cochrane Collaboration's Consumer Network website (http://www.informedhealthonline.org), with systematic reviews directed toward consumers of health care, is a wonderful site with funny cartoons that illustrate important concepts and some unexpected resource gems. For example, posted April, 2004, on that site was an article by Alessandro Liberati called "Meta-analysis: the science of analyzing groups of trials." For our readers who have spent many hours trying to learn about and teach meta-analysis, this article, directed toward consumers, was especially revealing of the very nonpaternalistic efforts of the Cochrane group to keep no "academic secrets" from patients. Very refreshing, eh?

WHY IS EBP SO IMPORTANT?

It really doesn't require much *logical reasoning* to see why EBP is so important. It just makes sense to base health practices on the best evidence because most of the time it costs less and almost all the time there are better patient outcomes. You'll note that we don't say it's always less expensive; sometimes the best approaches are costlier because they are newer. However, when we factor in costs of not practicing by evidence, the few times it costs more will be far outnumbered by the overall cost savings. What constitutes *better patient outcomes* must be clarified with caution—we must always take into account the patient's wishes, values, and so forth. Once in awhile, for all kinds of reasons, patients will refuse what providers see as the best evidence-supported approaches. Ultimately we must respect patient wishes as long as we know their decisions are based on the best available information. For more discussion on patients' roles in this thinking journey, look back to Chapter 6, "Patient-Centered Care."

CLINICIANS: ON WHAT IS YOUR PRACTICE BASED?

Before we launch into the thinking accompanying EBP, stop for a minute and think about your practice arena. Is your practice and that of clinicians around you based on knowledge you learned in school? How long ago was that? How many journals do you read? What drives you to read them? What determines when you consider a change in your practice? Does it come from you or from some outside source? How often do you search the Internet? For what topics? What are your sources of information?

Many clinicians will admit that they often do things because of past practice. Something stuck in their minds that worked. We are all very influenced by extreme events that stand out vividly in our memories—those where something very positive or very negative occurred. Nursing practice is often directed by such events. While learning from past peak experiences is important, there is danger in allowing those critical events to direct our practice too much, as you will see in TACTICS 8.1.

TACTICS 8.1: Clinicians, On What Evidence Do You Base Your Practice?

Reflect on these issues:

1. What, in your past, has been a "critical event" in your nursing practice? (Examples: A patient fell after you gave him a vaccination. A family became very upset when you told them the patient's blood pressure was slightly elevated. A patient started to yell very loudly when you touched her arm. A patient told you he could always breathe better after drinking a glass of cold water. A clogged PEG tube opened up miraculously when you flushed it with Coca Cola.)
2. Was it a positive or negative event?
3. When and under what circumstances did it occur?
4. How much has this event influenced how you practice in similar situations?

After answering those questions, go search for evidence to support or negate what you are doing in that area of practice. You may want to read the rest of this chapter and Chapter 9, "Critical Thinking and Informatics," before you start your search because we'll discuss the thinking that will help you with that search.

Discussion

Without reflection such as this, we can go merrily along without realizing what a tenuous basis there is for our actions. We have a saying that you've probably used yourself: "She's basing that conclusion on an N of one." The danger, of course, in basing actions on an "N of one" is that the event may have been a fluke. Flukes are definitely not part of EBP (except perhaps to fishermen? . . . Groan . . .). What worked well for one patient does not provide evidence for generalizing to other patients.

EDUCATORS: ON WHAT DO YOU BASE YOUR TEACHING?

Just as we've asked clinicians to reflect on their practice, so, too, we ask educators to consider the knowledge base they use for teaching. How old is it?

Are you teaching the most current evidence and are you encouraging your students to seek out the best evidence?

TACTICS 8.2: Educators, On What Evidence Do You Base Your Teaching?

How are you doing with promoting EBP? Look at your last teaching plan and answer these questions:

1. Am I handing down information or helping students seek knowledge?
2. How old is the information I'm using?
3. How many times do I use the word "evidence" or EBP?
4. Have I searched for the latest evidence on this topic?
5. If I searched, how did I evaluate the evidence I found?
6. Do any of my course objectives address EBP and thinking?

Discussion

While most educators would like to think they teach the most up-to-date information, it is very easy to get in a rut and use the same notes year after year. That can no longer be an option. If we expect clinicians to access and use the best evidence for practice, we need to teach them how to do just that. We need to demonstrate how we are finding and evaluating new information. In the next section that links CT with EBP, you will see how teaching can promote that thinking.

LINKS BETWEEN CRITICAL THINKING AND EBP

Look back to the beginning of this chapter (p. 145) to the four tasks set forth by the IOM as necessary to EBP. There are many such lists of tasks or steps to this process (for example, "Evidence-based clinical . . ." n.d.; Sackett, et al., 1997). Here is one posted on the University of Alberta's website:

- Identifying a problem or area of uncertainty
- Asking a relevant, focused, clinically important question that is answerable
- Selecting the most likely resources to search
- Searching and appraising the evidence found
- Assessing the clinical importance of the evidence
- Assessing the clinical applicability of the evidence
- Acting on and appropriately applying the evidence
- Assessing the outcomes of your actions
- Authoring-summarizing and storing records for future reference ("Introduction to . . . ", 2003, para 2)

As you can see, EBP is not simple; it's a set of complex tasks, all of which require CT. We have simplified the task list a little in Figure 8.1 in order to superimpose the thinking dimensions onto the components of EBP. Let's walk through that process. Look again at Figure 8.1 (on page 146) and start at the bold *Questioning Practice* point on the left.

Questioning Practice

This questioning is the absolute essential starting point on the path of EBP; one must approach healthcare and specifically nursing practice as a dynamic process that changes as our knowledge base grows and patients' situations change. The initial question might have to do with almost anything—an intervention, a specific patient population characteristic, a potential complication, an expected outcome or a specific task.

Inquisitiveness makes that questioning process come alive when clinicians wonder if they are practicing in the best possible way. Nurses who are eager to know and seek knowledge and understanding because they are naturally curious will more than likely seek the best knowledge/evidence all the time. They are the seekers of knowledge, not the takers. Seeking is an active process; taking is a passive process.

Intellectual integrity augments that inquisitiveness; nurses who value EBP will seek the truth of best practice evidence even when that questioning makes more work and increases discomfort as the status quo is shaken up. Nurses with strong *intellectual integrity* will give up traditional care approaches when there is strong evidence for changes in practice. An "N of one" will not be a legitimate source of evidence.

Another part of questioning practice is *intuition*. Think about nurses who have "gut feelings" that there must be a better way to do something. It's a fairly common phenomenon, often not acknowledged because, on the surface, it seems not to be part of EBP. However, those vague feelings that there should/ might be better approaches often drive nurses to go further, searching for those improved possibilities.

Evidence from Research and Other Valid Sources

Move to the next EBP task in Figure 8.1. Only after clinicians' questions become focused can they look for the best evidence to find answers. Although we have the CT dimension *discriminating* a little further along the path, clinicians definitely use it to help them hone the question. Remember our discussion of problem-based learning in Chapter 5—that focusing on a problem or question makes way for the exploration and learning that follows in this EBP process.

This search for best evidence is not simple. The best evidence doesn't magically appear in front of each clinician; there must be some effort at *information seeking*. In the old way of thinking, nurses practiced one way until a manager came along and handed out a new policy. Today, with EBP, there will be management-level mandates for change, but each individual nurse cannot wait for that information to be distributed to him/her. There is too much evidence appearing constantly. Nurses must individually and collectively promote *information seeking* to find the best practice standards. They must move beyond expecting to find answers in their immediate environments and learn how to find for themselves the best information from multiple sources.

This *information seeking* process seems, at first, very complex and may be overwhelming to nurses with limited backgrounds in research language and methods. However, increasingly there are excellent resources that offer assistance in how to find, analyze, and critique the quality of evidence (for example, Di Censo, Guyatt, & Ciliska, 2005; Melnyk & Fineout-Overholt, 2005). We also have lots of help from technology today as we do on-line searches for new evidence. We will discuss this more in Chapter 9, "Critical Thinking and Informatics," but for now, think about your abilities relative to search technologies. Have you done a CINAHL or MEDLINE search on a computer? Can you define a topic narrowly or broadly enough to be successful finding articles?

Despite the availability of computer searches and new technology, nurses must approach gathering evidence with their *analyzing* skills in top form. The process of searching for evidence requires that the question be broken down into manageable parts, the best search techniques must be sought and used and, when difficulties in finding evidence arise, the searcher must again turn to *analysis* to figure out how to break down the search problems further.

We're sure our readers have all done some searching for articles. Nevertheless, to illustrate this process let's look at an example: Say you're a nurse on a surgical floor and you're interested in decreasing post-op infections and finding the best way to do wound dressings. You could take a traditional approach to searching that you probably learned in school. Go to CINAHL and do a literature search. What words would you search under? We did just that by logging on to our university library, pulling up the CINAHL search engine, and typing in these subjects: "post operative wound care" and "nursing." Two-hundred-nine results came up, with article titles as diverse as "post operative pain" and "artificial nails." Using *analysis* to break things down more, we added a time frame of the past three years and the peer-reviewed criterion. Now 63 articles were listed. Subjects were still pretty diverse, such as "pressure ulcers post surgery" and "hearing loss post surgery." Nevertheless, we were able to scan through 63 titles, marking those that seemed to relate to wounds and operative procedures. After downloading and reading a couple of articles, we did not feel we had a good grasp on the body of evidence out there but we certainly were using our thinking dimensions of *information seeking* and *analysis*.

As an aside here, we need to note that we are assuming most readers have a working knowledge of the scientific research process and are able to recognize a research study and read it critically. It is obviously beyond the scope of this book to go into all of that. If our readers need to refresh that part of their knowledge, we recommend you review a research textbook.

Continuing with our example, our next step was to visit the Cochrane Library to see if they had done any systematic reviews of evidence related to post-operative infections. We'll discuss the thinking surrounding systematic reviews and then come back to this example again as we move through our critical thinking skills and habits of the mind.

Synthesis of Evidence (Systematic Reviews)

Fortunately, today there are many professional groups who collect research findings, do analyses, and compile syntheses of evidence bases—often called systematic reviews. Some of these sources we mentioned earlier— AHRQ, the Cochrane Collection, and Joanna Briggs Institute are popular examples—but the number of sources for evidence synthesis is growing rapidly. These groups are doing the time-consuming job of collecting all the evidence (articles and so forth), making judgments about the quality of that evidence, and compiling it into reports.

The Cochrane Collaboration is the largest organization producing and maintaining systematic reviews in health care right now (Clarke, 2003) and their library can be accessed by any organization with a subscription. In the Cochrane Collection we found, among others, for example, one systematic review on dressings and topical agents for surgical wounds (Vermeulen, Ubbink, Goossens, de Vos, & Legemate, 2004), and another on removal of nail polish and rings to prevent surgical infection (Arrowsmith, Maunder, Sargent, & Taylor, 2004).

So, where does that take us relative to EBP? Can we shut down our thinking a bit because we have found reviews by the prestigious Cochrane group? You know the answer to that must be "no" of course. Whether nurses are finding specific research reports or finding compilations of research (systematic reviews), those sources must be read with *discrimination*. Nurses must *analyze* reports and *discriminate* the quality of the evidence. There are standards to help clinicians do just that, and nurses are *applying standards* as they judge the quality of the evidence and the conclusions reached by those conducting reviews.

A very important part of understanding and *discriminating* systematic reviews is determining how the evidence was gathered and judged for strength.

There are standards that should have been applied and you need to look for them. Systematic reviews, if they are indeed "systematic," must report how the evidence was collected so that you, the reader, can judge whether it was thorough and systematic. Theoretically, you should be able to reproduce what they found by following the report of their search process. You must be able to see the strength of the evidence and how that strength was judged. The Cochrane Library has a reputation of excellence in doing reviews that is equalled by no other group (Clarke, 2003), so you might be able to trust their reviews a bit more than those of other organizations. Nevertheless, keep that keen *analytical* and *discriminating* ability in high gear at all times.

Now, how about the issue of "strength of evidence"? It used to be that this was a fairly simple issue, but that is changing today. There are debates over what constitutes legitimate and/or best evidence. Formerly we just listed some examples of evidence hierarchies. For example, Stetler et al. (1998) proposed this evidence hierarchy going from the best to the least-valued evidence:

I. Meta-analysis of multiple controlled studies

II. Individual experimental study

III. Quasi-experimental study

IV. Nonexperimental study (for example, descriptive, qualitative, case studies)

V. Systematically obtained, verifiable quality improvement program evaluation of case report data

VI. Opinions of nationally known authorities based on their experience or the opinions of an expert committee, including the interpretation of nonresearch-based information; regulatory or legal opinions

You will note that this hierarchy has meta-analysis of multiple controlled studies at the top. Many groups, such as the Cochrane Collaboration (Alderson, Green, & Higgins, 2004), have specified randomized controlled trials (RCT) as the gold standard for the best evidence. Recently, methods of judging evidence have been questioned because in some areas of practice we only have expert opinions and no research; also, there is a vast amount of research that is noncontrolled, descriptive, qualitative, and so forth. Caution in being too rigid is being advocated (Romyn, et al., 2003). Some nurses advocate revised hierarchies because there are few RCTs in nursing (Cesario, Morin, & Santa-Donato, 2002; "Evidence based nursing," 2004). Groups such as the Cochrane Collaboration, with stringent standards for "evidence" therefore include fewer nursing studies in their reviews.

Today we are seeing a lot more discussion of how to rate the strength of evidence, but we are not at the point where we have widely accepted standards. Right now, for example, the American Academy of Family Physicians has been working on a *Strength of Recommendation Taxonomy (SORT)* (Ebell, et al., 2004). AHRQ (2002, February) has been studying the issue intently. The 2004 Cochrane Reviewers' Handbook has this to say, while acknowledging that they focus primarily on systematic reviews of RCTs: "Systematic reviews of other types of evidence can also help those wanting to make better decisions about healthcare, particularly forms of care where RCTs have not been done and may not be possible or appropriate" (Alderson, Green, & Higgins, 2004, Section 1, Introduction, p. 13). Perhaps we will have more standardization by the time you read this; but more than likely, several approaches will remain for determining strength of evidence.

Ultimately, readers of systematic reviews must always look for criteria used to determine the strength of evidence. Because there are no hard and fast rules about what constitutes the "best" evidence, the reader's thinking is crucial. Readers must have *discriminating* abilities to see similarities and differences in the various studies and the conclusions about the body of evidence. They must look for and *apply standards* while thinking.

Evidence-Based Clinical Guidelines or Recommendations

Ultimately, because EBP is all about improving practice, clinicians need evidence translated into practice recommendations or clinical guidelines. Many groups that do systematic reviews go the next step and develop those guidelines. If you visit some of the websites in Box 8.2 on page 148, you will find lists of evidence-based clinical guidelines and/or links to other sites with guidelines. However, you can't turn off your brain when you find a guideline. You must use those thinking dimensions we discussed in the preceding section and add *logical reasoning.* All conclusions reached about what should be done in practice must be supported by the evidence. Indeed, when using prepared guidelines one should look to see if the trail from evidence to recommendations can be easily tracked.

There are many groups that offer criteria for evaluating clinical guidelines. We've compiled a list of them in Box 8.3 using the references we have included in that box. We recommend that our readers access The AGREE Collaboration project (2001) for a more comprehensive instrument that has been tested for validity and reliability (The AGREE Collaboration, 2003). One must never assume that guidelines are based on the best evidence, even if a seemingly trustworthy group developed them. We have to make our own judgments about how evidence-based they are. There is much potential for harm if guidelines

---

Box 8.3

Judging Clinical Practice Guidelines

- Is the guideline too vague to be usable?
- Is the guideline too specific to be practical with your patient group?
- Who developed the guideline?
- Are the developers qualified to develop this guideline?
- How broad is the representation of the group?
- Were healthcare consumers part of the group?
- Are there any potential conflicts of interest because of developers or sponsors of the guideline?
- Is there a clear explanation of the evidence used to develop the guideline?
- Is there an explanation of how the strength of evidence was determined?
- Could you retrieve the evidence easily?
- How strong is the evidence supporting the guideline's recommendations?
- What is the date of this guideline? Is it current?
- When was it last updated? Is there a reasonable pattern of updates?
- Has it been tested? By whom?
- Are there other guidelines available in the same area? If so, how consistent are they?

(Refs: Centre for Health Evidence, 2001; Grol et al., 1998; National Guideline Clearing House, n.d.; Shekelle et al., 1999; The AGREE Collaboration, 2001; Thomson et al., 1995.)

---

are used without their careful evaluation (Woolf, Grol, Hutchinson, Eccles, & Grimshaw, 1999).

Feasibility of Use with Patient Population

Once clinical guidelines are found or established, one must determine the feasibility and desirability of using those guidelines in a specific practice setting. This activity certainly requires a *contextual perspective*. One must consider the patient population, their preferences, and their values. One must consider the institution where the guidelines are to be used. How feasible is it to implement those guidelines? What resources are available for implementing it?

The Joanna Briggs Institute website (http://www.joannabriggs.edu.au) lists a set of questions to spur CT in considering applicability of evidence in clinical practice: "Is it available? Is it affordable? Is it applicable in the setting? Would the patient/client be a willing participant in the implementation of the intervention? Were the patients in the study or studies that provided the evidence sufficiently similar to your own to justify the implementation of this particular intervention? What will be the potential benefits for the patient? What will be the potential harms for the patient? Does this intervention allow for the individual patient's values and preferences?" ("Our history," n.d.)

Considering the feasibility of using evidence-based guidelines with specific patient groups is best done by those providers working directly with patients and by patients themselves. Academics cannot stand afar and say that certain guidelines must be used with all patients. People who know patients best should make these decisions. However, those folks must be educated about EBP and what constitutes good, better, and best evidence. This is one reason why the consumer focus of the Cochrane Collaboration (Clarke, 2003), for example, is so exciting. Not only are health providers knowledgeable about practice guidelines, now consumers can make better decisions.

Making decisions about feasibility of evidence-based guidelines accentuates the need for *all* providers and future providers to be educated about EBP and the various components of that process. And, most of all, they must realize the importance of CT as part of this process. Some might say that EBP is the antithesis of CT, reasoning that EBP means following the recommendations/guidelines that are formulated (often by groups outside one's personal arena) in cookbook fashion. Sackett, Rosenberg, Gray, Haynes, and Richardson (1996) responded to this best: "Evidence-based medicine is not "cook-book" medicine. Because it requires a bottom-up approach that integrates the best external evidence with individual clinical expertise and patient-choice, it cannot result in slavish, cook-book approaches to individual patient care" (para 6).

If, in the ideal world, we had evidence-based guidelines that appeared in front of us in a timely manner, even then there would be a need for the *contextual perspective* of CT. As with any "standardized" approach, such as assessment guidelines or clinical pathways, there will always be those who have an image of patient assembly lines and who just "do the job and go home." However, as most nurses realize, thankfully, the individuality of patients supercedes all such imagery and forces even the most slothful nurse to think. Evidence-based guidelines actually provide clinicians with tools that augment rather than impede CT.

Guideline Implementation Mechanism

Predicting as a CT skill is imperative as nurses move toward a specific plan or mechanism to implement evidence-based guidelines. As anyone who has promoted change will quickly tell you, this process also requires *creativity*. How do you get clinicians, educators and patients to value evidence-based guidelines enough to commit to implementing those guidelines? How do you devise a system easy enough to follow so that the system of implementation doesn't bog down? Sometimes it's as simple as thinking about the people who will be implementing the guideline and talking to them about the best mechanism.

Recently I attended a conference on EBP and one of the speakers was discussing such mechanisms. Being a gung-ho informatics advocate, I expected this educator to say that he was developing some elaborate plan for his medical students to download guidelines onto their PDAs. When I asked, he replied, "Oh no, I'm thinking along the lines of a laminated card for students and residents to carry in their pockets." It's hard to predict at this point in time, but maybe the old-fashioned approaches still work the best: because we are asking people to change what they do, maybe we will have more luck if we keep the mechanism of implementing that change simple.

Revision of Practice

Ultimately, if practice is to be revised to be consistent with best evidence, all those involved in the process must be *open-minded* and *flexible* in their thinking. The persons advocating the change in practice must not demoralize those who would prefer to hang on to tradition, but use *creativity* to help them increase their *flexibility*. This is, of course, no easy task. It is beyond the scope of this chapter and this book to describe all the dynamics of the change process but, certainly, anyone contemplating a true commitment to EBP will want to know all the nuances and strategies for successful change. We discuss the thinking involved in change in Chapter 11, "Thinking Realities of Yesterday, Today, and Tomorrow," but before we leave this subject we'd like you to reflect on your reaction to the last change proposed at your institution.

TACTICS 8.3: How Have You Reacted to Past Practice Changes?

Clinicians and Educators

Take a few minutes and think about a practice or teaching/curriculum change that you either supported or resisted—the ban on acrylic nails, moving IV flushes from heparin to saline, changing skills check-offs to a less rigid format, moving form sterile to clean techniques for dressings, and so on. Use these questions to guide your reflection.

1. Did I support this or not?
2. If I did, how did I show that support?
3. If I didn't, how did I react?

4. Were my comments and actions proactive or reactive?
5. Was my response emotional or based on my thinking?
6. How much knowledge did I have in making my decision to support or not support this?

Discussion

While we haven't talked much about the change process in this chapter, it is clear that approaching practice and education with an evidence-based perspective requires some change on our parts. It behooves us all to think about how we deal with change generally and how we deal with practice changes specifically.

Evaluation of Effectiveness of Change

Evaluating the effectiveness of a specific change of practice based on evidence is very important. Besides showing us if this was a good move, the evaluation process reminds us to continue questioning practice. We should no more go on our way thinking a new approach to practice allows us to rest on our laurels than we should continue blindly doing what we've always done. We must critically evaluate what's been done and how it can be done even better.

Judging the effectiveness of a change requires planning ahead (*predicting*) to determine important data to collect and for how long. It requires *logical reasoning* as one makes conclusions about this change. The skeptics will sit up and take notice when we can show, with objective data, why this change saved money, increased patient satisfaction, decreased complications or length of stay, and so forth.

Back to the Whole Picture of CT and EBP

EBP is not for the faint-hearted. That's why CT *confidence* is written across the bottom of Figure 8.1 as the "*sine qua non*" of this process. Hopefully you have developed *confidence* in your thinking skills as you have learned to embrace EBP. There are three other CT dimensions that cross over and are used through the entire EBP process, and those are *transforming knowledge, reflection,* and *perseverance.*

EBP **is** *transforming knowledge*: The whole EBP process is the quintessential example of that CT skill. We are taking evidence and adapting and adopting it to our uses. EBP is also a process of *reflection* at each stop along the way. One must constantly reflect on practice, the need for change, the change process, the results of the change, and so forth. And, as anyone who has tried to do nursing with an EBP approach, *perseverance* in one's thinking processes is also essential. There will certainly be obstacles, some big and some small, depending on how large a change is required based on the evidence available. Ultimately, while the picture of the interrelationships of the CT components and the components of EBP might look like a neat oval process, it is of course not that clean, nor are the "steps" mutually exclusive.

BIG, SMALL, INDIVIDUAL, AND GROUP MOVES TOWARD EBP

As we have been discussing EBP so far, aside from our little foray into searching for information on post-op wound care, we have not specified examples of EBP in action. Individual nurses can move to EBP as a daily way of thinking and/or can focus on moving their teams in that direction. It is certainly ideal to work with a team who values EBP. That group will share evidence they find; they will plan changes together and support each other in the process. We often think that CT is an individual phenomenon, but look at the thinking points in Figure 8.1 from the perspective of your group. And then, if you're really brave, keep your EBP hat on and look at it from the perspective of Interdisciplinary Teams as described in Chapter 7.

Now, consider EBP in terms of magnitude. Sometimes a major change in policies and procedures is called for as we get new evidence. Take, for example, the recent strong evidence that tight control of glucose post op for cardiac patients drastically reduces sternal infections (Clement et al., 2004; American College of Endocrinology, 2004). Many institutions are working on new protocols for glucose control via IV insulin. Here in Michigan, for example, Marcia Hegstad, Clinical Nurse Specialist for Diabetes at a large teaching hospital, has done extensive work with an interdisciplinary team to develop guidelines for physicians and nurses to follow based on this evidence (personal communication, Marcia Hegstad, July 20, 2004). That change in practice has been hugely effective in reducing the incidence of sternal infections post-cardiac surgery. Extensive interdisciplinary team thinking went into that EBP area. Look at Chapter 11 for more details of Marcia's story.

Here's an example of a smaller nature—one nurse with an EBP mindset. Imagine this scenario: A nursing assistant on an adult medical-surgical unit takes vital signs on all patients. Nurse A glances at the results, sees nothing very far above 140/90 (the traditional "normal"), tells the aide to record them and goes on with the day. Now, using *analysis* and a *contextual perspective*, Nurse B might think about the data as they related to the specific patient, evaluating the normalcy of each reading.

If Nurse B is using EBP, the diabetic patient with a blood pressure of 140/90 will stand out as in need of attention because that nurse will be aware of the best evidence to direct practice. The American Diabetes Association (2004) in their recommendations for hypertension management in diabetics used strong research evidence from the UK Prospective Diabetes Study (UKPDS) (The Oxford Center, n.d., American Diabetes Association, 2004) showing that for each 10-mmHg decrease in systolic BP there was a 12% decrease in risks for any complication, 15% for diabetes-related death, 11% for MI, and 13% for micro-vascular complications. Citing the UKPDS and other strong evidence, the American Diabetes Association (ADA) developed guidelines (easily available on their website, http://www.diabetes.org) recommending that blood pressures of less than 130/80 be maintained for diabetics (ADA, 2004).

Any nurse working with diabetics—and these days that includes virtually all nurses—must vow to keep abreast of the enormous body of diabetes research evidence that has exploded over the past few years. Fortunately, groups such as the ADA continually review that research systematically and translate the evidence into clinical guidelines that are reviewed and updated yearly. All guidelines are freely available on the ADA website. Nevertheless, there are many clinicians working with diabetics who continue to practice with only traditional information. We should question why that is so.

In the above example, we used the critical thinking skill of *analyzing* and the habit of the mind, *contextual perspective*, to illustrate a first step toward EBP. However, nurses in similar situations would need to use far more CT skills and habits to fully accomplish a goal of EBP. As we discussed earlier, two of the most important habits of the mind to promote those early steps toward EBP are *inquisitiveness* and *intellectual integrity*.

TACTICS 8.4: Clinical Practice "Question of the Month"

Clinicians

Try this on your unit: Each month, create a contest for the best clinical practice question. Encourage nurses to search for guidelines or evidence to support or negate usual practice and post them in a specific place such as the gathering room. Rewards can be whatever is the most coveted thing in that group—time off, money for conferences, a new uniform, or "chits" that can be saved and turned in for things such as being taken off the float list for six months. Such behavior could be built into evaluation criteria.

Take that a step further and post criteria for evaluating the strength of evidence of a summary report or a clinical guideline. (Consider using the AGREE instrument described earlier.) Have a contest for who can most accurately judge the strength of evidence for changing practice. If you want to really take it further, have them identify the thinking skills and habits of the mind used in this activity.

Educators

Use the same strategy with students. Whatever course you're teaching, build into your syllabus credit for students formulating questions about practice, finding the latest evidence, evaluating it, and discussing if and how that evidence should be used.

Discussion

As educators, we have used this tactic to teach EBP principles. In our nursing research classes we have students write their major paper on a clinical issue that they explore for the latest evidence. They show their knowledge of the research process in discussing the evidence they found. Box 8.4 has several other general suggestions for activities to promote EBP both in clinical and classroom situations. Hopefully they will help you think of specific TACTICS that will work for you.

ONE NURSE'S STORY OF SUCCESSFUL EBP

Before we end this chapter we'd like to share this story. Judy Meyers is a Clinical Nurse Specialist in Gerontology, who has successfully cultivated EBP on her in-patient unit at a large teaching hospital here in Michigan (personal

---

Box 8.4

Suggestions for Promoting EBP in Clinical and Classroom Settings

- Incorporate reflection activities into assignments that require thinking about EBP
- Have students or nurses work in groups to do an EBP activity of their choice and identify how the 17 dimensions of CT were used in that activity.
- Create an EBP Tracking Thinking Diagram modeled after Figure 8.1 or let students create one.
- Build EBP expectations into evaluation criteria for promotions or grades.
- Make a list of how you can socialize a group to emphasize not only EBP but the underlying thinking skills needed to operationalize EBP.

communication, Judy Meyers, July 19, 2004). She has, over the past few years, instituted changes in several areas of practice: use of fewer indwelling foley catheters, a protocol to assess and treat agitation, decreasing the number of orders for bed rest, liberalized diets for the elderly, an activity project to get older people up and moving. She is now working on a plan to improve nurse–physician communication. Here are some excerpts of our conversation, especially those where she revealed her thinking as she planned and instituted these innovations. You will also note that she makes reference (without prompting, we might add) not only to EBP, but also to the other four IOM competencies: interdisciplinary practice, patient-centered care, quality improvement, and use of informatics.

TACTICS 8.5: Find the Thinking and the Five IOM Competencies in Judy's Story

Clinicians and Educators

As you read the story below, take a pen and circle the parts that illustrate thinking dimensions and the five IOM competencies.

I knew the problems caused by foley catheters and so many of our patients had them. I prepared a self-learning module for the nursing staff on bowel and bladder management for older people and, in the bladder part, discussed reasons why you don't want indwelling catheters. I did a literature review and a proposal to change our policy. I found the CDC guidelines for judging when foleys are necessary and, along with Dr. Alan Dengiz, a Geriatrician, we developed a protocol outlining the CDC criteria and 4 others that we added, such as terminal illness, severe perineal excoriation, etc.

We educated the physicians. I went to the Medical Section meeting to get the support of all the department heads and they took the information back to their peers. Most of them were in favor of the protocol. We put the protocol into the computer for nurses to follow. They could assess patients and discontinue catheters without waiting for an order from an MD.

In another example, I noticed that we had a lot of patients with orders for bed rest. I worked with physicians on this and tried to get them to understand that this was bad. We audited charts for 3 months to check how many patients had orders for bed rest or bathroom privileges only. We found the older patients were, the more likely they were to have those orders; 52% of patients over 70 had an initial order for bed rest. When questioned, the physicians said they were ordering bed rest because they didn't know what the patient could do.

I did a review of literature and took a proposal to the MDs. I worked with people in electronic data entry and had them take out "bed rest" that was at the top of the order options, put it at the bottom with a required write-in section for the reason to justify the bed rest order. We also added an option to d/c bed rest. The percentage of patients with bed rest orders went from 52% to 5%; those who have the orders have things like hip fractures so those orders are appropriate.

I'm always thinking what do our patients need? What do we need to be doing better? If I notice something I collect data. If you want MDs to buy into something, you need data. I check the literature and I let staff know what I find. They are much more apt to go along with something if they can see why we should be doing it, especially if it's an uncomfortable thing. I think ahead to what's going to be difficult in doing this. I make things as easy as possible. I educate staff, go out and role model what I'm talking about and I specifically work with people who are resistant.

I also have a great nurse manager who is good at creating the expectations of quality. She is right there in the thick of things. She is committed to excellent care and needs to be doing what is state of the art. She goes to conferences and brings ideas back to me.

Right now we're working on improving nurse/physician communication. Physicians want nurses to give concise, pertinent information; they want nurses to know the patients well. Nurses tend to use narrative approaches and focus on relationships. Some physicians come on the floor and leave without ever talking to a nurse; nurses have to call them more frequently than they should. Right now I'm doing a review of the literature on this subject and planning a quality improvement project for this fall. We'll start small and most of the initiatives will come from nurses. One idea is to have laminated cards for nurses to use when calling physicians; those cards would have reminders of important information to include in their reports. Another is to institute MD/RN rounds to facilitate sharing information.

Physician Geriatricians tend to be EBP advocates. For example, several years ago one of them saw a bladder scan used in a nursing home and asked me if we could look into getting one. We did and now every unit in the hospital has one. We did it first. One of the biggest aids to EBP is constant curiosity.

Discussion

We'll bet many of you would like to work with Judy. Are you fortunate enough to work with nurses like her? Are you a nurse like her? She exemplifies EBP, doesn't she?

PAUSE AND PONDER:
WHERE SHOULD OUR EBP THINKING GO?

OK, so you're totally convinced that EBP is the bandwagon you should be on, right? We hope you can approach this not as a bandwagon, but as a way of thinking for excellence in practice. It is a more enlightened and exciting approach that gets us away from tradition as a driving force. However, it is changing very fast and we must be clear on what we are promoting when we say EBP. As Estabrooks (2003) cautioned, there is a lot of jargon—"research utilization, knowledge utilization, innovation diffusion, technology transfer, evidence-based practice, knowledge translation, knowledge transfer and knowledge mobilization . . ." (p. 62). It is all about using the best knowledge we have for practice and that knowledge will not just be handed down. It must be sought actively. Recognizing when we need it, accessing it, evaluating it, using it, and evaluating its usefulness is a constant cycle requiring CT.

Reflection Cues

- EBP is an important paradigm shift away from practice based on tradition to one based on use of the best knowledge available.
- The IOM envisioned EBP as several tasks—knowing where and how to find best evidence, formulating clinical questions, searching for and evaluating the evidence to answer those questions, and determining how and when to integrate that evidence in practice.
- EBP requires the use of all 17 dimensions of CT.
- The history of EBP shows an international movement that primarily started in the 1980s and continues today.
- There is increasing focus on health consumers' part in the EBP movement.
- EBP is important because most of the time it saves money and other resources and promotes better patient outcomes.
- Clinicians and educators need to reflect on how they use evidence in their daily work.
- Links between CT and EBP can be easily tracked.
- Questioning practice is augmented by *inquisitiveness, intellectual integrity,* and *intuition.*
- Searching for evidence necessitates the use of informatics and the thinking dimensions of *discriminating, information seeking,* and *analysis.*

- Synthesis of evidence in systematic reviews is done by several groups today, notably the Cochrane Collaboration.
- Users of systematic reviews must evaluate them with *discrimination*, use *analyzing*, and *apply standards* for judging quality.
- Mechanisms to judge strength of evidence are currently being studied extensively.
- Using evidence-based clinical guidelines requires *logical reasoning* so that recommendations for practice can be traced back to the evidence.
- A *contextual perspective* is imperative when considering the feasibility of using evidence-based guidelines with patient populations.
- EBP is not cookbook healthcare.
- Implementing EBP requires *predictive* thinking and *creativity*.
- Revising practice is best done with *open-minded, flexible* thinking.
- Evaluating effectiveness of practice changes requires *logical reasoning* and *predicting*.
- The whole process of EBP requires *confidence* in one's thinking, *reflection*, and *perseverance*.
- EBP is a process of *transforming knowledge*.
- EBP can be done with large innovations or in small, day-to-day increments.
- One nurse's story about how she is using EBP helps us appreciate how this is possible and how important CT is to this process.
- Clinicians and educators must take care not to approach EBP with a bandwagon mentality, but with CT fully engaged.

References

Agency for Healthcare Research and Quality (2002, February). *What is AHRQ?* Rockville, MD: Author. (AHRQ Pub. No. 02-0011). Retrieved August 6, 2004, from http://www.ahrq.gov/about/whatis.htm.

Agency for Healthcare Research and Quality (2002, April). *Fact Sheet: Rating the strength of scientific research findings.* Rockville, MD: Author. (AHRQ Pub. No. 02-P022).

Alderson, P., Green, S., & Higgins, J. P. T., editors. *Cochrane Reviewers' Handbook 4/2/2* [updated March 2004]. Retrieved July 18, 2004, from http://www.cochrane.org/resources/handbook/hbook.htm.

American College of Endocrinology Task Force on Inpatient Diabetes and Metabolic Control (2004). American College of Endocrinology position statement on inpatient diabetes and metabolic control. [Electronic Version] *Endocrine Practice, 10* (1), 77–82.

American Diabetes Association (2004). Hypertension management in adults with diabetes. *Diabetes Care, 27*, Supplement I, S65–S67.

Arrowsmith, V. A., Maunder, J. A., Sargent, R. J., & Taylor, R. (2004). Removal of nail polish and finger rings to prevent surgical infection (Cochrane Review). In: *The Cochrane Library*, Issue 2, 2004. Chichester, UK: John Wiley & Sons, Ltd. Retrieved July 18, 2004, from http://212.49.218.200/newgenMB/ASP/printDocument.asp.

Centre for Health Evidence (2001). *Users' guides to evidence-based practice*. Retrieved June 24, 2004, from http://www.cche.net/usersguides/guideline.asp.

Cesario, S., Morin, K., & Santa-Donato, A. (2002). Evaluating the level of evidence of qualitative research. [Electronic version] *Journal of Obstetric, Gynecologic, and Neonatal Nursing, 31* (6), 531–538.

Clarke, M. (2003, August). *The Cochrane Collaboration*. Retrieved June 24, 2004, from http://www.informedhealthonline.org/item.aspx?tabid=20&pagerequest=3.

Clement, S., Braithwaite, S. S., Magee, M. F., Ahmann, A., Smith, E. P., Schafer, R. G., & Hirsch, I. B. (2004). Management of diabetes and hyperglycemia in hospitals. *Diabetes Care, 27* (2), 553–591.

Di Censo, A., Guyatt, G., & Ciliska, D. (2005). *Evidence-Based Nursing: A Guide to Clinical Practice*. St. Louis: Elsevier Mosby.

Driever, M. J. (2002). Are evidence-based practice and best practice the same? *Western Journal of Nursing Research, 24* (5), 591–597.

Ebell, M. H., Siwek, J., Weiss, B. D., Woolf, S. H., Susman, J., Ewigman, B. & Bowman, M. (2004). Strength of recommendation taxonomy (SORT): A patient-centered approach to grading evidence in the medical literature. *American Family Physician, 69* (3), 548-556. [Electronic version.]

Estabrooks, C. A. (2003). Translating research into practice: Implications for organizations and administrators. *Canadian Journal of Nursing Research, 35* (3), 53–68.

Evidence-based clinical practice working group (EBCP) (n.d.). Retrieved June 24, 2004, from http://www.fhs.mcmaster.ca/ceb/acts/ebcp.htm.

Evidence based nursing (University of Minnesota), Retrieved June 24, 2004 from http://evidence.ahc.umn.edu/ebn.htm.

Evidence-based practice centers (n.d.). Retrieved August 6, 2004, from http://www.ahrq.gov/clinic/epc/.

Grol, R., Dalhuijsen, J., in't Veld, C., Rutten, G., & Mokkink, H. (1998). Attributes of clinical guidelines that influence use of guidelines in general practice: observational study. *BMJ, 317*, 858–861.

Haller, K. B., Reynolds, M. A. & Horsley, J. A. (1979). Developing research-based innovation protocols: Process, criteria and issues. *Research in Nursing and Health, 2*, 45–51.

Higgs, J., Burn, A., & Jones, M. (2001). Integrating clinical reasoning and evidence-based practice. *AACN Clinical Issues, 12* (4), 482–490.

Introduction to evidence based medicine (2003, April). Retrieved June 24, 2004, from http://www.med.ualberta.ca/ebm/ebmintro.htm.

Institute of Medicine (2003). *Health professions education: A bridge to quality*. Washington, DC: The National Academies Press.

Jennings, B. M. & Loan, L. A. (2001). Misconceptions among nurses about evidence-based practice. *Journal of Nursing Scholarship, 33* (2), 121–126.

Liberati, A. (2004, April). *Meta-analysis: The science of analyzing groups of trials*. Retrieved June 24, 2004, from http://www.informedhealthonline.org/item.aspx?tabid=26&pagerequest=2.

Melnyk, B. M. & Fineout-Overholt, E. (2005). *Evidence-based practice in nursing & healthcare: A guide to best practice*. Philadelphia: Lippincott Williams & Wilkins.

National Guideline Clearinghouse. (n.d). *Guideline comparison description*. Retrieved August 6, 2004, from http://www.guidelines.gov/about/GuidelineComparisonDescrip.aspx.

Our history (n.d.). Retrieved July 17, 2004 from: http://www.joannabriggs.edu.au/about/history.php.

Profetto-McGrath, J., Hesketh, K. L., Lang, S., & Estabrooks, C. A. (2003) A study of critical thinking and research utilization among nurses. *Western Journal of Nursing Research, 25* (3), 322–337.

Romyn, D. M., Allen, M. N., Boschma, G., Duncan, S. M., Edgecombe, N., Jensen, L. A. et al. (2003). The notion of evidence in evidence-based practice by the nursing philosophy working group. *Journal of Professional Nursing, 19* (4), 184–188.

Sackett, D. L., Rosenberg, W. M. C., Gray, J. A. M., Haynes, R. B, & Richardson, W. S. (1996). Evidence-based medicine: What it is and what it isn't. (Article based on editorial from the *British Medical Journal, 312,* 71–72.) Retrieved June 24, 2004, from http://www.cebm.net/ebm_is_isnt.asp.

Sackett, D. L., Richardson, W. S., Rosenberg, W. & Haynes, R. B. (1997). *Evidence-based medicine: How to practice & teach EBM.* New York: Churchill Livingstone.

Sams, L. & Gannon, M. E. (2000). Evidence-based practice and clinical work assessment. *Seminars in Perioperative Nursing, 9* (3), 125–132.

Shekelle, P. G., Woolf, S. H., Eccles, M., & Grimshaw, J. (1999). Developing guidelines. *BMJ, 318,* 593–596.

Stetler, C. B., Brunell, M., Giuliano, K. K., Morsi, D., Prince, L. & Newell-Stokes, V. (1998). Evidence-based practice and the role of nursing leadership. *JONA, 28* (7/8), 45–53.

The AGREE Collaboration (2001). *Appraisal of guidelines for research & evaluation: AGREE instrument.* Retrieved August 6, 2004, from http://www.agreecollaboration.org.

The AGREE Collaboration (2003). Development and validation of an international appraisal instrument for assessing the quality of clinical practice guidelines: The AGREE project. *Quality & Safety in Health Care, 12,* 18–23.

The Oxford Centre for Diabetes, Endocrinology & Metabolism (n.d.) *UK Prospective Diabetes Study.* Retrieved August 6, 2004, from http://www.dtu.ox.uk/ukpds/results.html.

The name behind the Cochrane Collaboration. Retrieved June 24, 2004, from http://www.cochrane.org/docs/archieco.htm.

Thomson, R., Lavendere, M., & Madhok, R. (1995). Fortnightly review: How to ensure that guidelines are effective. *BMJ, 311,* 237–242.

Vermeulen, H., Ubbink, D., Goossens, A., de Vos, R., & Legemate, D. (2004). Dressings and topical agents for surgical wounds healing by secondary intention (Cochrane Review). In: *The Cochrane Library,* Issue 2, 2004. Chichester, UK: John Wiley & Sons, Ltd. Retrieved May 7, 2004, from http://212.49.218.200/newgenMB/ASP/printDocument.asp.

White, P. J. (2002). Evidence-based medicine for consumers: A role for the Cochrane Collaboration. *Journal of the Medical Library Association, 90* (2), 218–222.

Woolf, S., Grol, R., Hutchinson, A., Eccles, M., & Grimshaw, J. (1999). Potential benefits, limitations, and harms of clinical guidelines. *BMJ, 318,* 527–530.

Youngblut, J. M. & Brooten, D. (2001). Evidence-based nursing practice: Why is it important? *AACN Clinical Issues, 12* (4), 468–476.

CHAPTER 9

Critical Thinking and Informatics

The computer, the telephone, the Web, video—these, and all that is still to come, are unquestionably powerful tools. Used badly, they waste time and money, and dehumanize our interactions with each other. Used well, guided by a clear understanding of basic informatics principles, they are neither to be feared, loved nor loathed. They are simply to be used. In the next century, the study of informatics will become as fundamental to the practice of medicine as anatomy has been to the last.

That poignant statement is from Enrico Coiera's paper, based on an article he wrote for the *Medical Journal of Australia* in 1998 and posted on the Internet as *10 Essential Clinical Informatics Skills* (n.d.). He is referring to informatics—a term that is now as much a part of nursing and healthcare delivery as the bedpan. While it is commonplace, informatics is not a natural subject for most nurses; however, it is being thrust upon us as a necessity because computer technology and the information it processes are here to stay.

Health informatics is about how we process, use, and share information relative to healthcare delivery. The Institute of Medicine (IOM), with its conjoint emphasis on patient-centered care, evidence-based practice, quality improvement, and interdisciplinary practice, described the competency of utilizing informatics as "communicate, manage knowledge, mitigate error, and support decision making using information technology" (2003, p. 46).

Clearly evident in that definition and Coiera's statement is that critical thinking (CT) needs to be an integral part of using informatics. Coiera's 10 skills almost all start with words that imply thinking—"understand," "search for and assess," "interpret," "analyze and structure clinical decisions," "adapt and apply knowledge," "access," "assess," "select and apply," "structure and record data," and so forth. The IOM statement includes "manage knowledge" and "support decision-making." Using informatics has great potential; it will require a whole lot of thinking, but it will improve our thinking, too. CT's relationship with informatics will be this chapter's focus.

THE CONTEXT OF OLD NURSES AND YOUNG INFORMATICS

Some of you may be tempted to skip this chapter because you think you won't understand informatics. Maybe it's something you're just not interested in.

You probably get really angry at all the cell phone conversations in restaurants and stores and the exorbitant prices you pay for cable TV and computer games for your teenagers. Stick with us and you'll see you are not alone in your frustration over informatics. We sympathize with you on a personal as well as professional level because we're also "old" nurses dealing with "young" informatics.

If you remember when we didn't use computers every day, you are possibly our age. When we started out in nursing in the late '60s and early '70s computers were props in science fiction movies—big, cumbersome things that filled whole buildings, whirring and whizzing to help the spies. Thirty-some years later we're unable to imagine life without these machines—now small as peas—that we love and hate. (Yes, Dr. Coiera, in spite of what you say, we do love and hate them.) We love them because they make access to information so easy. We hate them because when they freeze, flash blue screen messages, lose our last three hours of writing, get viruses, and other situations too numerous to list, we are left with the realization that we are way too dependent on them. For most of us that dependency is scary because so much of today's technology is mysterious. The one thing we all know, though, is that information technology is here to stay and it's evolving more rapidly than we can fathom.

Those of us in the baby-boom generations have lived through the birth and rapid growth of computers. We've learned this foreign language later in life. For several years, we wrote with a pen and then typed things into the computer—the old typewriter mentality. (Don't worry; we've grown up; we're now typing original ideas here sans yellow pad.) We oldsters have had to change our ways to keep up with computers. For younger generations, computers are as common as electricity was for most of us back then. However, many nurses are our age and older. The average age of nursing faculty today is 51.2 years (American Association of Colleges of Nursing, 2003). (Arrrrrrrgh!) The average age of the working nurse is 43.3 years, with RNs under 30 representing only 10% of our ranks (National League for Nursing, 2004). The majority of nurses did not grow up with computers in their homes; many used a computer for the first time in their places of employment. Many still anxiously stumble along using computers every day.

Almost everyone around us uses computers in some way—if not directly, at least indirectly. In Chapter 6 we discussed patients surfing the Internet to find out things such as what medications they want, the best treatment options, and current standards of care. Consumers of healthcare have more access to information than they have ever had before. People who think they can survive in this world without integrating informatics into their lives are dinosaurs trying to survive in the 21st century. We're getting ahead of ourselves here, but we wanted to show you that reading this chapter is worth the effort, even though it may be scary to your middle-aged eyes. We apologize to our youthful readers but, according to the statistics, you are a minority. Let's go back and set up more groundwork.

HEALTHCARE INFORMATICS EVOLUTION

Lest we lead you down a confusing path, and before we join CT with informatics, we'll detour here to discuss the evolution of health informatics more. It used to be that informatics meant computer technology, and so far we have focused many of our comments in that direction. Because computers were the instigators of this field, we often equate them with informatics. Today, however, the focus of this burgeoning field is more on information. The UK Health Informatics Society website (2004) noted that we are ready to change from a focus on computers and technology to stressing meanings of information in communicating, sharing knowledge, and decision making.

As you may deduce from that statement, not everyone defines informatics in the same way. The term "informatics," coined in the 1970s, initially referred to computers and their immediate context (Saba, 2001). Since that time, people have broadened descriptions, some doing it according to discipline. For example, "nursing informatics" according to Saba and McCormick (2001) is:

> The use of technology and/or a computer system to . . . process . . . and communicate timely data and information in and across health care facilities that administer nursing services and resources, manage the delivery of patient and nursing care, link research resources and findings to nursing practice, and apply educational resources to nursing education (p. 226).

The American Medical Informatics Association, on its website, acknowledges that "medical informatics" shares some common ground with other healthcare specialties, but asserts that medical informatics has its own emphasis. They defined medical informatics as having ". . . to do with all aspects of understanding and promoting the effective organization, analysis, management, and use of information in health care" (n.d.).

There are debates about informatics being discipline-specific, i.e. medical informatics vs. nursing informatics (Masys, Brennan, Ozbolt, Corn, & Shortliffe, 2000). We have broader, interdisciplinary definitions such as biomedical informatics (Columbia University, n.d.) and, recently, adding to the terminology conundrum are the terms "patient informatics" (for example, Bader & Braude, 1998; Williams, Gish, Giuse, Sathe, & Carrell, 2001) and "consumer health informatics" (for example, Eysenbach & Jadad, 2001).

The British folks, in what seems like a common-sense move, have adopted the term "health informatics." The UK Health Informatics Society (formerly the British Medical Informatics Society) had what seems to be the most straightforward but comprehensive interdisciplinary description of health informatics on their website: "[Health informatics] . . . can be best understood as the understanding, skills and tools that enable the sharing and use of information to deliver healthcare and promote health" (n.d., para 1). They noted that the term "health informatics" is replacing the term "medical informatics." The broader term, focused on health, allows all healthcare disciplines and patients to be part of this important field.

Clearly evident from these various descriptions is that informatics has to do with managing information/knowledge, communicating, and making decisions—all direct links to thinking. The IOM specifically pointed out its value in preventing errors, which fits with their emphasis on increased safety in healthcare. The subject of safety and reducing errors in healthcare is addressed more in the next chapter.

The Changing Nature of Informatics

In considering how to approach the subject of CT and informatics, we were struck with the real probability that anything we said about informatics would be out of date by the time this book was published. Indeed, as one reads about informatics one can readily see that, unless informatics information has been

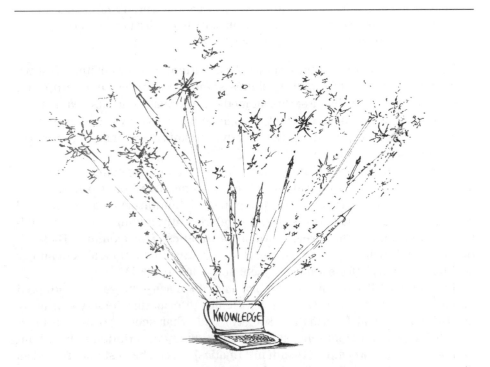

Knowledge Explosion

posted on a website in the past six months, it is out of date. This rapid rate of change, of course, is due to the increasing sophistication of the technology we use to share and use information.

We're trying to get a feel for where informatics will be going in the near future, but by the time we sit down to write that, the future has become the present. Nevertheless, we'll try to keep as much of a "futuristic" view as possible in our comments about CT and informatics. The IOM in its latest Quality Chasm Series, *Patient Safety* (2004), is calling for three important foci for informatics that can contribute to increased quality in healthcare. They are proposing increased support from government agencies and healthcare systems to accelerate improvement of: a) data exchange formats, b) structured terminologies, and c) knowledge representation. These three areas will facilitate recording and accessibility of information, increase the intersystem and interdiscipline communication, and facilitate decision making. For example, the IOM (2004) would like to see the Agency for Healthcare Research and Quality (AHRQ), National Institutes of Health (NIH), Food and Drug Administration (FDA), and similar agencies support the development of generic clinical guideline models in computer-executable formats to help with evidence-based practice and clinical decision support. You will recall from Chapter 8 that implementation of clinical guidelines is still a challenge, largely due to inadequate mechanisms to ease their use in daily practice.

Another interesting view of the present and near future of informatics was articulated by Ball and Lillis. Even though they published this in 2000, which by informatics standards is very old, their observations about trends remain relevant. Using information from the Gartner Group Research Review, Ball and Lillis (2000) discussed eight trends in healthcare information technology. Those eight are paraphrased in Box 9.1.

As you look at the box you can probably see yourself in the middle of those trends right now, maybe even past them. The constant, rapid rate of change of informatics and our panting alongside to keep up ultimately are reasons why addressing the thinking involved in informatics is so critical. All healthcare providers need to have a CT frame to go along with the rapid changes. That thinking frame will have built into it ways of dealing with the changes in those mechanisms that can enhance our thinking. That thinking cannot be linear or dualistic; it must be contextual and relativistic. Thinkers who are uncomfortable with uncertainty will either give up or they will suffer extreme stress.

CRITICAL THINKING AND HEALTH INFORMATICS

The merger of CT and informatics comes from two directions. As seen in Figure 9.1, one can augment one's CT with informatics but one must use CT to

---

Box 9.1

Eight Trends in Health Care Information Technology
(Ball & Lillis, 2000)

1. *Data to decisions:* technology will automate more decision-making processes. (For example, decision trees or algorithms.)
2. *Communication to collaboration:* there will be more knowledge sharing across cultures and geography will become irrelevant.
3. *Information to knowledge:* information will be more integrated via technology. (For example, Internet vs. books; e-mail vs. snail mail.)
4. *Network computing to ubiquitous computing:* specifically where the information is stored or processed will become unimportant. (For example, desktop computers to laptops to PDAs to pocket whatevers.)
5. *Graphical to cognitive user interfaces:* technologies such as speech recognition and natural language processing will enhance ease of using technology. (This will dramatically change the nature and speed of dictation into medical records, for example.)
6. *Situated to mobile:* we will need to meet the needs of people on the move and in remote locations. (Imagine this example: You work at a small rural center but you can link to larger facilities easily.)
7. *Physical to virtual:* technologies such as "smart cards" and "e-commerce" will make things simpler. (I can't wait for my virtual colonoscopy, can you?)
8. *Business to customer:* we will need to consider the needs of users beyond our immediate environment.

---

best choose and use informatics. Informatics is only slightly akin to a new piece of equipment (for example, needle-less needles) that, once mastered, can be used to augment work. Informatics include many processes, changing daily, that are there for our use if we know enough about them and are open-minded enough to choose them.

In Figure 9.1 we have listed several CT dimensions on the left side that help us choose and use informatics. The list on the right side indicates the dimensions augmented by informatics. There is some overlap of those dimensions and we will address the reasons for that overlap shortly. You will also note that we have the dimension of *transforming knowledge* up at the top with health informatics and *reflection* as the connecting dimension with the arrow at the bottom. Why have we done that?

Figure 9.1   Relationship Between Critical Thinking and Health Informatics

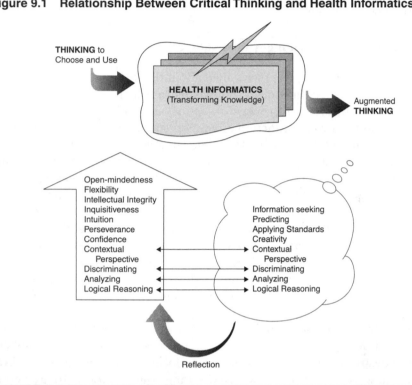

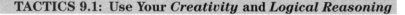

TACTICS 9.1: Use Your *Creativity* and *Logical Reasoning*

Clinicians and Educators

Before reading further, stop a minute and look at Figure 9.1 and reflect on the 17 CT dimensions that we have revisited frequently throughout this book. Test your creative thinking and logical reasoning to consider why we might have placed the dimensions where we did.

Discussion

The next section will give you our explanation, but this TACTICS encourages you to construct your own meanings first. Then compare to see if you thought of things that we forgot. It's quite possible that you put all 17 dimensions on both sides. As you realize by now, artificially separating CT dimensions is just that—artificial. In reality we use all dimensions in most thinking situations. What we've done here is try to tease out those that are especially important to each side of the picture. Rest assured, there are other ways to interpret this; you may have come up with a much different configuration.

Informatics as Transforming Knowledge

Earlier (remember Dewey?) we talked about the difference between information and knowledge. Informatics allows us to transform information into knowledge and allows us to *transform knowledge*—change or convert the condition, nature, form, or function of concepts among contexts. That's why we have highlighted *transforming knowledge* in Figure 9.1.

Consider a computer application used by a nurse practitioner for prescribing medications. In the old days, the practitioner would have to consider other medications the patient was taking and try to think if there were any potential interactions. She would spend time looking up such things and there would be a good chance something would be missed because there were several places that could, and should, be checked. Today, when using a program like *epocrates.com*, for example, information on each drug is made available so that, in one fell swoop, all potential interactions are noted, dosing for certain conditions listed, and so on. The drug information has been transformed into usable knowledge and in a very timely manner.

How about a staffing example? In the old days, doing staffing plans by hand meant long hours of figuring out numbers and acuity of patients on units at various times of the day, week, or month and then projecting needs accordingly. There were lots of places where thinking could go awry. Today's computer programs can transform all the information we give them into patterns that tell us with a greater degree of certainty what our staffing needs will be.

The very act of communicating within an informatics framework allows for the transformation of knowledge much more easily. Let's take a really simple example: writing on a computer as opposed to writing on a typewriter or a pad of paper. Anyone who writes as we do—stream of consciousness first and then moving things around and editing next—will definitely say that transforming information and knowledge is so much easier on a computer. You get the idea, right? Using informatics *is transforming knowledge*—sorting it, analyzing it, communicating it, and converting it into a practical, usable form.

CT for Choosing and Using Informatics

At the left side of Figure 9.1 eleven CT dimensions are listed that are particularly used to choose and use informatics. The last four in the list (*contextual perspective, discriminating, analyzing,* and *logical reasoning*) are repeated on the right side of the figure because, in addition to helping thinkers choose and use informatics, those dimensions also are augmented by informatics. Those will be discussed here and in the section entitled "How Informatics Augments CT" later in this chapter, on page 187.

Open-mindedness and Flexibility

First and foremost are the *open-mindedness* and *flexibility* CT dimensions. Using informatics means changing from how one has been doing things before—either using applications for the first time or keeping up with newer applications. We'll bet many of you can remember, as we do, the first year we moved our teaching materials over to PowerPoint programs. It seemed like such a big deal, and it would have been so much easier to stick with our handwritten notes and overhead transparencies. Today we expect PowerPoint presentations and are shocked when someone doesn't use them. Maintaining a *flexible* and *open-minded* approach to new methods of gathering, storing, sorting, *analyzing*, and using information is a challenge because we seem to always be at the start of a learning curve.

Intellectual Integrity

Related to *open-mindedness* and *flexibility* is *intellectual integrity*—seeking the truth even when it goes against one's assumptions and beliefs. This is a tough one because it is so much easier to maintain the status quo: "The way I do things now works just fine"; "I don't want to learn a new way"; "I don't have time or energy." We've all said those things, especially on a Friday after a long week.

Just how does one maintain an *open mind*, the *flexibility*, and the *intellectual integrity* to embrace informatics? For starters, it helps to receive positive reinforcement for those thinking habits of the mind. Second, it's important to tell yourself that you can't survive in this field without informatics. (You can't, you know; it's definitely a force to be reckoned with.) Third, start talking about informatics to the people you work with and with those who work at institutions like yours. Ask them what they know, their visions, fears, and reality when it comes to information technology. Fourth, make yourself sit down at a computer and do something you've not done before. To get you started with those four suggestions, try TACTICS 9.2.

TACTICS 9.2: Think How Informatics Could Ease Your Life

Clinicians and Educators

Take some time and reflect on informatics and then think about your daily activities. Even if you know nothing about computers or information technology, where do you think you could improve your job efficiency and accuracy with technology? Don't allow yourself to think about the specifics of changing over to such technology; that will shut down the open-minded side of your brain. Be a divergent thinker; let your thoughts expand!

Discussion

What did you come up with? Did you let your creative juices flow? As clinicians, we'd want voice-activated recording devices, hand-held computer "terminals" that we could put in our pockets to access and record information. We'd want all patients to have a "smart card" with their health data on it—one that we could insert into our hand-held device and retrieve and record information. Perhaps, by the time you're reading this book, you'll laugh because you have such devices with you. Maybe you'll laugh even more because what you have goes far beyond our old-fashioned vision.

As educators, we would want teaching aids that "talk" to each other more easily. We'd want instant, sure-fire Internet access in every classroom. We also would want those hand-held devices that we can carry around and use easily. We'd want functioning virtual classrooms where people can talk to each other around the world, all at the same time. We'd want students to have these hand-held resources where, if they have to do tracheostomy care, they can pull up a virtual demonstration anytime and anywhere. You get the idea, right? Let your mind soar; almost anything our limited minds can envision will most likely be a reality very soon.

Inquisitiveness

Getting back to our dimensions for choosing and using informatics, it will help your *intellectual integrity* if you engage your *inquisitiveness* habit of the mind. Are you naturally inquisitive? If so, you've probably already explored the various information technologies available to you. If you are less inquisitive, try to tweak it more—but do it with fun activities. For example, go to the video store and get some movies that deal with informatics—not necessarily science-fiction stuff, but stories about people who are touched by technology. If you need suggestions, here are some examples (in no particular order) listed by Tyler, one of our sons who is a movie buff: *Jumping Jack Flash, Being There, The Conversation, Blow Out, Apollo 13, Enemy of the State, The Net, Eternal Sunshine of the Spotless Mind, You've Got Mail, Something the Lord Made,* and *Wag the Dog.*

Need more suggestions to get your inquisitiveness going? Get a computer program that's fun—a game or drawing program that you can really "get into."

Talk to kids about technology. Consider where you are first, though—that could scare you off because kids are really knowledgeable; they grew up with this stuff. Find the person in your environment you secretly call the "techno-geek" and strike up a conversation about why s/he is so into technology. Go on the Internet and look up people you know; you may be surprised what you find. Try to find friends from your past whom you've lost track of. Write e-mails to those persons. One of us, because of a simple e-mail request, has had a wonderful renewed friendship with a childhood friend with whom she was out of touch for 30 years. The point of these activities is to immerse yourself in technology and information exchange. It's hard to be inquisitive about something that you've never played around with.

Intuition

Intuition can help enhance one's choosing and using informatics. That may seem a bit strange at first glance because *intuition* seems so subjective and informatics seems so objective, but it really isn't that dichotomous. Computers can't be *intuitive* but we can be. Without *intuition* we won't be able to use technology, including computers, as well as we could. Just because the computer program dictates that we do something a certain way doesn't necessarily mean it's the best or only thing to do in that situation. If it doesn't feel right, chances are it isn't.

To illustrate more subtle connections between intuition and informatics, let's get away from computers and use a simple, more familiar technology example: Your patient needs an injection of enoxaparin; it comes from the pharmacy in its syringe—technical aids to your work. You double-check the dose (*applying standards*) and you go to administer it. How do you know how much pressure to use when you inject the short needle? Can you remember the first time you gave a sub-cutaneous injection? You may have not punctured the skin or did it so hard you were almost past the hub. What guides you to know how much pressure to exert? That doesn't come from the instrument. Effken (2001) would call that "prospective control"—*intuitive* visual information. That information is so taken for granted by experts that many would not call it thinking. Because *intuition* usually comes with experience, and because most of us are new to informatics, it's easy to forget about *intuition*. With repeated use of informatics and openness to "gut" responses, we allow *intuition* to help our CT.

Perseverance

Perseverance is an absolute necessity for using informatics, especially if this field is new to you. Recently, in one of our early classes on evidence-based practice, students complained about the amount of time they spent searching the In-

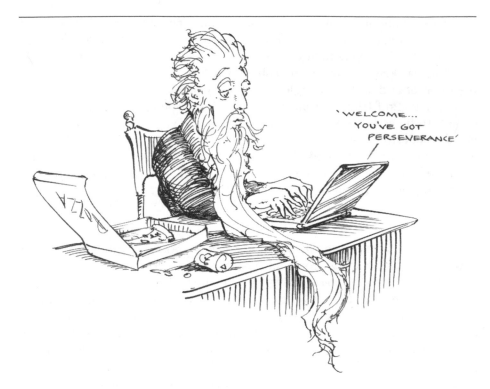

ternet to find the evidence reports they needed. They had horror stories of spending hours in one area, only to discover they could have saved that time if they had gone to another website first. Some students gave up, thinking eight hours on the computer was excessive. Many were surprised when we didn't bat an eyelash and they heard similar stories from their classmates. We discussed the realities of time when using new technologies and how important *perseverance* was, especially in doing something new like evidence searches.

In our old ways of getting information—asking someone, finding a book, searching library index cards—there were fewer options for search paths. Less *perseverance* was needed to think from question to answer. Today we "noodle" around on the computer/Web for hours before finding what we're looking for. (That's our favorite description—"noodle"—implying that this is not a straight, linear process.) Because we are new to computers and their mechanisms to address information, we are slower than we think we should be.

It's an interesting position to be in—most nursing leaders, as noted at the start of this chapter, were not raised in homes where computers were commonplace. We are learning a new language and a new set of skills constantly. Because we are experts in our fields already, we have trouble accepting the fact that, when it comes to today's technology, we are just novices. Look at teenagers and young adults today—they can maneuver around a computer program so fast that we're left in the dust. We take much longer to do everything because it's still so new to us. We often say we don't have enough RAM to do things fast. (You can tell how in-the-know about computers your listeners are when they either laugh or don't at that remark.) We must maintain *perseverance* and accept our novice status relative to informatics.

Confidence

Related to our novice technophile status is *confidence*. It is hard to have *confidence* in one's thinking in unfamiliar territory. This is an area where it is helpful to separate *confidence* in doing something from *confidence* in one's thinking ability. We can accept our novice states and the reality of our clumsiness and anxiety when using new information technology, but still have *confidence* in our abilities to think. Actually, the latter will help the former. A *confident* thinker can often figure out unknown computer commands just by relying on his/her own logic. Computers are, in spite of what we think sometime, very logical. However, they don't "think" as such; they only follow our commands or the commands of the programmer. In that area we are superior. Having a little sign over your desk that says "Computers can't think but I can" is helpful to *confidence*-building.

We should not underestimate the negative effects of anxiety on our thinking *confidence*, however. If you are choosing and directing the implementation of a new technology for your work unit, for example, consider how you might decrease the anxiety of the staff as they begin this difficult process. First and foremost, we must acknowledge the negative effects of anxiety on thinking and that working with a new technology produces anxiety. There is nothing more anxiety-producing than to anticipate looking stupid. We tend to respond in anger and use pretty low-level thinking skills. Let's get that on the table and acknowledge we're all in that boat when we try something new.

Second, we must set up support services. Nurses take pride in their self-sufficiency; we have strong thinking skills and manage on our own quite well. Well, it's time to swallow that pride and accept the fact that we all need help with informatics. A technology or informatics expert should be available at all times to staff using something new. That person should be in place before the initiation of a new system.

Along that same line, we need to broaden our view of our teams when we increase our use of informatics. One thing we say to our students frequently is "the librarian is your friend." We forget, as we set out to do things such as finding evidence-based clinical guidelines or what computer programs are available for our consideration, that librarians are expert in such searches. Older people (we) often have this old-fashioned view of librarians as bespectacled, quiet people who stamp and sort books. Well, wake up and get rid of that view. Have you talked to librarians recently, especially those with a specialty in healthcare informatics? They are phenomenal resources and we need an updated vision of who they are and how they can be critical to our use of informatics. Crumley and Koufogiannakis (2002) listed six domains of librarianship. Three of those six are providing service and access to information; helping users with library resources; and creating better methods to retrieve and access information. ". . . The librarian's role has expanded to include the role of teacher or consultant as well as that of expert mediated searches" (Calabretta, 2002, p. 34).

TACTICS 9.3: Take Your Librarian to Lunch

Clinicians and Educators

OK, this may seem a bit hokey but bear with us here. If you know your librarian well and s/he often helps you, then you probably can skip this TACTIC. But, if you've never thought of your institution's librarian in Calabretta's terms (above), go to the library, send an e-mail, or call the librarian and ask that person to lunch with you. Tell him/her that you would like to pick his/her brain about health informatics.

Discussion

If you did this, we'll bet you were pleasantly surprised in terms of what you learned about that person's knowledge and willingness to help you. You will feel more confident in your thinking relative to informatics once you know you have this resource. You may also find someone who would be delighted to come to your unit or classroom to help with informatics.

Contextual Perspective

We have now arrived at the four dimensions that are on both sides of Figure 9.1. *Contextual perspective* is a thinking habit of the mind that is important to choosing and using informatics, and it is augmented by informatics. Here we focus on the choosing and using part: If you are the person choosing computer applications for your office or unit, for example, you need to think about the whole picture. Who will be using them? What will they cost? Which are easy to use? What will they add to or subtract from your resources? Take time to explore all possibilities.

Keep in mind that, just as they aren't *intuitive*, computers are noncontextual; however, we have to use them with a *contextual perspective*. If you are using a staffing program that says you need a staff of 10 people for Saturday, it will not tell you to think about the forecasted sunny day and the big party someone is having (factors that might very well influence how many call-ins you have). If the computer tells you each practitioner should be able to see four patients every hour, you can't be a slave to that; you must look at the context of who those patients are (sometimes older people take 5 of their 15 minutes just to walk back to the exam room).

Discriminating

Another thinking dimension that will be augmented by informatics is also needed for choosing and using informatics: it is *discrimination*. One of the biggest drawbacks to information technology is the issue of reliability. Anyone can post anything on the Internet. They can identify themselves by any title. There is very little discrimination as to quality. This is a problem for all of us, but particularly for patients who may make health decisions based on indiscriminate information.

Some attempts are being made to remedy this for health consumers today. For example, the National Library of Medicine has lists of reliable health-related resources (http://medlineplus.gov). You can find several others in Box 9.2. Most of these websites have links to many others that they have checked

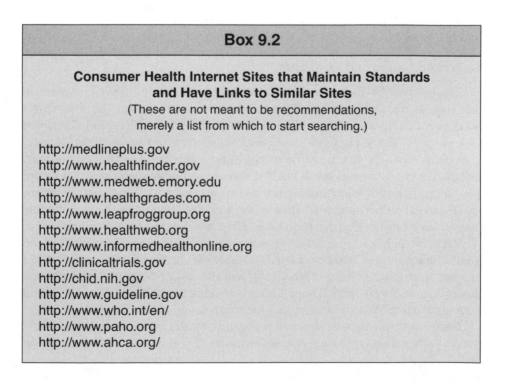

Box 9.2

**Consumer Health Internet Sites that Maintain Standards
and Have Links to Similar Sites**
(These are not meant to be recommendations,
merely a list from which to start searching.)

http://medlineplus.gov
http://www.healthfinder.gov
http://www.medweb.emory.edu
http://www.healthgrades.com
http://www.leapfroggroup.org
http://www.healthweb.org
http://www.informedhealthonline.org
http://clinicaltrials.gov
http://chid.nih.gov
http://www.guideline.gov
http://www.who.int/en/
http://www.paho.org
http://www.ahca.org/

out. However, a word of caution about using any website in a list in a book. They can change quickly, disappear, move, and so forth.

For healthcare providers looking for evidence-based clinical guidelines, you will recall from Chapter 8 that we suggested evaluation criteria for *discriminating* quality. Keeping such things in mind is very important as you exercise your *discrimination* thinking skills. You must constantly question what you see and read. You must also educate patients to be *discriminatory* in their thinking. People who have limited knowledge of a subject have more difficulty *discriminating* relative importance or validity of information. Walji et al. (2004) made a startling discovery when they analyzed 150 websites on alternative medicine: Thirty-eight sites (25%) had statements that could cause harm if acted upon; 145 sites (97%) had omitted information. Walji et al. (2004) cautioned consumers to use other means of validation of information found on websites.

In another example, a clinician recently told this story: A depressed patient was started on Lexapro and stopped taking it within two days because she felt worse. When the clinician questioned this, the patient said, "Well, I went on their website and it said this drug may worsen depression, so I figured that's what was happening to me." What the patient didn't do was read further to see the remainder of the explanation of how this drug's action builds. This example may remind you of a discussion in Chapter 6 and what we said about our responsibilities to help patients develop their CT skills.

Logical Reasoning and *Analyzing*

The last two CT dimensions on both sides of Figure 9.1, *logical reasoning* and *analyzing*, are augmented by informatics and used for the nitty-gritty work of choosing and using informatics. Get away from looking at informatics as a whole—a scary, big field—and break things down (*analyze*) into manageable units. If you're in a position of choosing a new information technology, ask these types of questions: What is it you are trying to accomplish? How are you doing it now? What's available as an alternative? What resources are needed to get something new? How will it work? What will be the surrounding issues? How long will a transition take? What are the costs and benefits?

If a new technology is thrust upon you, ask these questions: What is the goal of this change? What do I need to know? What do I know already that I can use during this change? How long will this take? Why am I angry? How anxiety-producing is this? What about it is making me anxious? How can I deal with my anxiety? Who and what do I have as resources?

Logical reasoning will help you make the best decisions, ones based on evidence rather than emotional responses alone. If you've come to a conclusion that a new technology forced on you by your manager is a bad idea, on what have you based that conclusion? If you're gung-ho to have a particular e-mail system in your institution, on what is your enthusiasm based? It's easy to be critical or overly enamored of new technology if we don't know much about it. Knowledge is power; not having knowledge about something thrust upon us makes us feel powerless and potentially frustrated in our actions. (Should we start looking for a new entry in the DSM-IV-TR: "Informatics Rage"? ☺)

How Informatics Augments CT

There is no question that, when used well, informatics can significantly help our thinking. Let's look at the CT dimensions listed on the right side of Figure 9.1. We'll start with the four we just discussed that are listed both on the left and the right sides—those that are both augmented by and necessary to choose and use informatics (*contextual perspective, discriminating, analyzing*, and *logical reasoning*). Then we'll discuss the four listed at the top (*information seeking, predicting, applying standards*, and *creativity*).

Contextual Perspective

The communication ability that is afforded by informatics has broadened our *contextual perspective* enormously. The Internet has broadened our patients' perspectives, but we don't yet have enough research to determine the full effect (Murray et al., 2003). While the system is still not without wrinkles, such as liability, confidentiality, and payment, some providers are using e-mail with patients (Patt, Houston, Jenckes, Sands & Ford, 2003; Forkner-Dunn, 2003). According to Forkner-Dunn (2003), about 100 million Americans obtained health information from the Web in 2002. They can broaden their resources by e-connecting with others who have the same medical conditions.

Discriminating

Not only does informatics broaden our contextual perspectives and those of patients, it also helps us with our *discrimination* of information. Remember, as we discussed in the section above, you also need sharp *discrimination* skills to use informatics. Now we're focused on how informatics can help that cognitive skill. We can access much more information and broaden our field so much that we can see patterns and differences in information. We can have computers link information for us to see if patterns exist; as educators we can predict where our students will have trouble with NCLEX exams by looking at patterns in their other tests. We can *discriminate* any list of things according to rank with the touch of one button.

Analyzing

It is easy to miss the forest for the trees and vice versa with our natural cognitive abilities and emotions. Informatics allows for ease of *analyzing*—breaking things down into manageable units. We're going to veer off a bit here with *analyzing* and look at it relative to standardized language. Computers require standardized descriptors of phenomena for programming. To standardize anything, one must break it down and give it a consistent designation (name, number, and so forth). Informatics has forced and helped nursing to define itself—to *analyze* the parts of our profession and standardize our nomenclature. These taxonomies have become standard—Nursing Diagnoses (NANDA), Nursing Interventions (NIC), and Nursing Outcomes (NOC).

Back in the 1970s, when the first talk of describing components of nursing according to nursing diagnoses began, it was triggered by the need for us to keep up with informatics. The first conference to classify nursing diagnosis was called in 1973 by two nurses from St. Louis, Gebbie and Lavin, for two reasons. One reason was related to clinical issues and the other was that they had been "offered space on a computerized record-keeping system" (Gordon, 1982, p. 2). You can't put something into a computer that has several names and definitions. It must be specific and broken down clearly. This need to specifically define our profession in terms of our diagnoses, interventions, and outcomes has already, and will continue to, benefit nursing. We transform data into nursing knowledge and build our theoretical frameworks in the field (Bakken & Constantino, 2001).

Look at the first chapter of the latest edition of the *Nursing Interventions Classification* (Dochterman & Bulechek, 2004) and you will see the long list of information systems that endorse its use; it is licensed for inclusion in the Systematized Nomenclature of Medicine, for example. Look at the *Nursing Outcomes Classification* (Moorhead, Johnson, & Maas, 2004) and you'll see a similar focus on this classification fitting into information systems; for example, it meets the American Nurses Association Standards from the Nursing Information and Data Set Evaluation Center. This need for a specific classification that can work with the systematic nature of information technology has been a large driving force for nurses in defining their discipline.

Logical Reasoning

Just as analyzing is both necessary for choosing and using informatics and augmented by informatics, so too is *logical reasoning* significant on both sides of the picture. Human *logic* of course is always influenced by emotions. We see things that don't necessarily exist because we want to see them. We ignore things in front of us because we don't want them to influence our decisions. Computers don't have that emotional component (except in some movies, like HAL in *2001: A Space Odyssey*). A computer can only deal with what's been put into it. Any "conclusion" reached by the computer is less likely to be influenced by human bias (taking into account the programmer); it has a *logical* progression back to the raw data put into it. While we must acknowledge the value of *contextual perspective* and *intuition*, those cannot stand alone if we are to be safe, effective, and efficient providers. The *logic* that informatics promotes is the balance for our human biases.

Information Seeking

Probably the easiest benefit to see from informatics is in *information seeking*. It's hard to imagine how we wrote papers and books before electronic searches, isn't it? You can find something about almost any subject on the Internet: You can access libraries around the world, and you can ask a question of someone in Taiwan as easily as you can ask it of the person in the office next door—sometimes easier. In terms of information seeking and access, we in our 50s frequently are in awe of this new ability we have. Of course, as we discussed earlier, *information seeking* without *discriminating* skills can be very problematic.

Predicting

Because of the help we can get with our *information seeking* and *discriminating*, we are also better at the cognitive skill of *predicting*. Because informatics allows us to see patterns, it is easier to *predict* how patterns will continue. Think about the move to prospective reimbursement (Beyers, 1985) if you need an "in-your-face" example of the *predictive* capabilities of informatics. Setting up the diagnostic related groups for prospective reimbursement was a method of *predicting* how long patients would stay in the hospital based on certain diagnosis-related data that were *analyzed* by a computer program. Budget programs help us *predict* what we'll need for the future. Computer scheduling applications help us *predict* how many nurses we'll need for the Saturday shifts in the summer. Tracking medication errors helps us *predict* problem medications as well as relationships between things like acuity or time of year and medication errors.

Applying Standards

Applying standards is sort of related to the earlier discussion of standardized language. In the same way that labels for nursing diagnoses, interventions, and outcomes are specified in information systems so that we're all on the same wavelength, so, too, can professional standards be unified and easily available.

To avoid being duplicative, we remind you to go or think back to the previous chapter on evidence-based practice. Our ability to access evidence-based clinical guidelines is justification enough that informatics helps with *applying standards*. We can practice with the best, most current standards because technology allows their availability to all clinicians. Joining a list-serve gives us nearly immediate updates without even having to search. Faculty can *apply standards* in their teaching by accessing the best information on their teaching topics. We can find all kinds of help with teaching methodologies in informatics. Standards to protect human subjects in research situations can be easily accessed through government websites.

Imagine yourself as a clinician on a hospital unit; you have to use an intervention you haven't done in a long time. In the old days, you could ask other nurses and possibly get the best standard of care or you could go through the policy and procedure manual—that dog-eared book in the conference room whose updates were often nebulous. In most institutions today you can pull up a computer program and find just what you need.

Creativity

Because we have tools such as computers at our fingertips, informatics can help our *creativity* thinking habits. Ask artists how their tools affect *creativity* and most will say that those tools augment their *creativity*. It is easier to be *creative* and individualize your patient teaching, for example, if you have videotapes, computer-based learning modules, and written materials to work with. If you are an educator, are you using those options to be the most *creative* thinker and teacher?

TACTICS 9.4: Using Informatics to Improve Teaching Creativity

Educators

Reflect on your teaching methods. When was the last time you updated them? Do an inventory of the available informatics that you may not be using to spice up your teaching.

Clinicians

Do a mental inventory of the things you repeatedly teach patients. Are you using standardized materials? Is it the most current information?

How many options are available to you to teach that material? Are you using the most efficient method to teach? The most creative ones? Have you used informatics to help you with this?

Discussion

Creativity is not something we think of as a companion to informatics because one seems so right-brain and the other so left-brain. However, when you think of informatics as a tool what it has to offer is boundless.

Reflection on CT and Health Informatics

We have now covered all the CT dimensions on the left and right sides of Figure 9.1. Obviously, dividing CT dimensions is somewhat false and awkward. However, keep in mind that you have to use CT with informatics and you also augment CT with informatics. It is time now to reflect on how it all fits together.

Reflection is the big arrow at the bottom of Figure 9.1. It's down there to remind you that there's nothing static about thinking when it comes to incorporating informatics in healthcare. You will constantly need to *reflect* on where you're going. As we have said many times now, informatics is constantly changing. While your thinking processes will be in these same 17 dimensions, you will need to keep all the doors and windows of your mind open to let in the new ideas and seize the new opportunities that informatics has to offer. You will always use *logical reasoning*, for example, but the data you have available to make decisions will certainly change. You will always need *perseverance* because unfamiliar pieces of informatics that you have to slog through will keep cropping up. A friend of ours likes to say "get over it" when people voice disgruntled opinions about the rapid change of technology. Your thinking will *persevere* because it will have to.

An overarching *reflection* focus is to be open to the future of informatics. According to Ball and Lillis (2000), whose trends we cited at the start of this chapter, new technology goes through three phases: replication, innovation, and transformation. Healthcare is lagging behind other systems, such as banking and airlines, in that it's still between the first and second phases. The first, replication, is where a manual job is replaced by a machine and the second, innovation, is a new way of doing something. The last phase, transformation, where an industry is completely transformed by informatics, has not yet occurred in healthcare. Ball and Lillis (2000) projected the three most important emerging technologies in healthcare to be ". . . the computer-based patient record (CPR), Internet/intranet/extranet applications, and clinical decision support (CDS) systems" (p. 389).

Just since the publication of the Ball and Lillis article, there have been great strides in CPR, but we are still a distance away from the full implementation of CPRs that can be used at the bedside with voice activation. Most institutions use Internet and intranet communication applications, but there are still many issues to deal with, such as patient privacy issues, before these are widely used by patients and providers. CDS systems are also not yet widely used. As those of us who live and breathe topics like critical thinking are quick to point out, the nuances and complexities of human decision-making can be augmented by computers, but we don't see how computers will replace that thinking. We might have telephone, e-mail, voicemail, or video mail available, but we still need a caring, thinking person to decide which one is best to use.

CHALLENGES OF INFORMATICS

There are many challenges facing us in healthcare and many of them can be helped with informatics. Critically thinking clinicians and educators must try to predict those challenges and how to overcome them. One of the frequently cited challenges is, of course, the cost of innovative technologies. Even though many of them will ultimately save large amounts of money, there is still an enormous outlay of resources to get new and better systems going.

Another issue is the human factor in accepting, choosing, and using informatics. We have several times touched on the difficulties folks in our age group have with informatics. Ironically, because of our age, we are leaders in our professions and therefore, we are making decisions about informatics. There are no simple answers to choices about informatics. That's why we must rely on our CT.

Repeatedly we see the need to work on quality evaluation tools for consumers of electronic information. Health search improvements, especially consumer-directed tools, are strong themes in Greenberg, Andrea, and Lorence's online health action agenda (2004). We need not only research in these areas, but also to develop education models for finding and intelligently using information.

Health professions are moving to meet these challenges. Specialists in informatics are increasing rapidly. The American Medical Informatics Association (AMIA), formed in 1990, has 3,200 members composed of physicians, nurses, computer and information scientists, biomedical engineers, medical librarians, researchers, and educators. It has among its working groups one for nursing and one for consumers ("About AMIA," n.d.) Canada's Health Informatics Association has 900 members from many health disciplines, including nursing (COACH, 2004).

Since 2000, there has been an eHealth Code of Ethics with this vision statement: ". . . to ensure that people worldwide can confidently and with full understanding of known risks realise [sic] the potential of the Internet in managing their own health and the health of this in their care" (eHealth Code, n.d., first para).

PAUSE AND PONDER:
HEALTH INFORMATICS AND THE FUTURE

We'll leave you with one parting challenge to consider: dare we even envision a healthcare future without a wholehearted embrace of informatics? Probably not, but neither should we embrace it without sharp thinking to determine the best technology and the best uses of it. For a sobering consideration, read Eysenbach's 2003 article on severe acute respiratory syndrome (SARS) and population health technology. This physician from Toronto General Hospital outlined the many technologies used both to help the crisis and to negatively fuel fear during the 2002–03 outbreak of this scary, new, deadly disease. Eysenbach cautioned us to learn lessons for future public health emergencies:

> Population health technology clearly has a vast potential to increase our preparedness for the next public-health emergency, but it also raises many questions related to ethics, libertarian values, and privacy, and has the potential to fuel an epidemic of fear and collective mass hysteria. (last para)

Reflection Cues

- Informatics has to do with managing information/knowledge, communicating, and making decisions.
- There are clear links between CT and health informatics.
- Healthcare technology is a vast, constantly changing force to be reckoned with.
- For baby-boom generation healthcare workers, informatics does not come as easily as it does and will for generations who grew up with computers.
- Healthcare informatics has been defined by discipline—e.g., medicine and nursing—but today there is a move toward the interdisciplinary idea of health informatics.
- Almost anything said to describe the current state of informatics in a textbook is out of date by the time the book is published; that's how fast things are changing.
- Having a futuristic perspective is helpful when considering informatics and the thinking surrounding it.
- Informatics is moving from data to decisions, communication to collaboration, information to knowledge, networking to ubiquitous com-

puting, graphical to cognitive user interfaces, situated to mobile, physical to virtual, and business to consumer.

- The relationship between thinking and informatics comes from two directions; one's thinking will be augmented by informatics but one needs CT to choose and use informatics.
- Informatics is a process of *transforming knowledge*.
- The primary CT dimensions needed for choosing and using informatics are *open-mindedness, flexibility, intellectual integrity, inquisitiveness, contextual perspective, intuition, perseverance, confidence, logical reasoning, analyzing,* and *discriminating*.
- Informatics particularly augments these CT dimensions: *information seeking, contextual perspective, discrimination, predicting, logical reasoning, analyzing, applying standards,* and *creativity*.
- *Reflection* is the CT dimension that must always be used to study where we are and where we're going with informatics.
- Computer-based patient records, Internet/intranet applications, and clinical decision support are three areas where emerging technologies are particularly active today.
- Challenges of informatics today are costs, human acceptance factors, and the need for better tools to judge quality of information.
- We have organizations such as AMIA and COACH and an eHealth Code of Ethics to meet some challenges.
- An important challenge is to embrace the rapid advances of informatics without doing it blindly and without ignoring quality, ethics, and values.

References

About AMIA (n.d.) Retrieved August 4, 2004, from http://www.amia.org/about/about.html.

American Association of Colleges of Nursing (2003). *Annual state of the schools 2002–2003.* Washington, DC: Author.

American Medical Informatics Association (n.d.). "History of Medical Informatics." Retrieved July 11, 2004, from: http://www.amia.org/history/what.html.

Bader, S. A. & Braude, R. M. (1998). "Patient Informatics": Creating new partnerships in medical decision making. *Academic Medicine,* 73, 408–411.

Bakken, S. & Constantino, M. (2001). Standardized terminologies and integrated information systems: Building blocks for transforming data into nursing knowledge. In J. M. Dochterman and H. K. Grace, *Current issues in nursing* (6th ed) (pp. 52–59). St. Louis: Mosby.

Ball, M. J. & Lillis, J. C. (2000). Health information systems: Challenges for the 21st century. *AACN Clinical Issues,* 11, 386–395.

Beyers, M. (Ed.) (1985). *Perspectives on prospective payment: Challenges and opportunities for nurses.* Rockville, MD: Aspen.

Calabretta, N. (2002). Consumer-driven, patient-centered health care in the age of electronic information. *Journal of the Medical Library Association, 90* (1), 32–37.

COACH: Canada's health informatics association (2004). Retrieved July 12, 2004, from http://www.coachorg.com/Default.asp?id=367.

Coiera, E. *10 Essential Clinical Informatics Skills.* Retrieved July 12, 2004, from http://www.informatics-review.com/thoughts/skills.html.

Columbia University Biomedical Informatics (n.d.). Retrieved July 11, 2004, from http://www.dbmi.columbia.edu/.

Crumley, E. & Koufogiannakis, D. (2002). Developing evidence-based librarianship: Practical steps for implementation. *Health Information and Libraries Journal, 19,* 61–70.

Dochterman, J. M. & Bulechek, G. M. (Eds.) (2004). *Nursing interventions classification (NIC),* 4th ed. St. Louis: Mosby.

Effken, J. A. (2001). Informational basis for expert intuition. *Journal of Advanced Nursing, 34* (2), 246–255.

eHealth Code of Ethics (n.d.). Retrieved July 17, 2004, from http://www.ihealthcoalition.org/ethics/ehcode.html.

Eysenbach, G. (2003). SARS and population health technology. *Journal of Medical Internet Research, 5* (2), e14. Retrieved July 14, 2004, from http://www.jmir.org/2003/2/e14/index.htm.

Eysenbach, G. & Jadad, A. R. (2001). Evidence-based patient choice and consumer health informatics in the Internet age. *Journal of Medical Internet Research, 3* (2), e19. Retrieved August 3, 2004, from http://www.jmir.org/2001/2/e19/index.htm.

Forkner-Dunn, J. (2003) Internet-based patient self-care: The next generation of health care delivery. *Journal of Medical Internet Research, 5* (2), e8. Retrieved July 14, 2004, from http://www.jmir.org/2003/2/e8/index.htm.

Gordon, M. (1982). Historical perspective: The National Conference Group for Classification of Nursing Diagnoses (1978, 1980). In M. J. Kim & D. A. Moritz (Eds.) *Classification of nursing diagnoses: Proceedings of the third and fourth national conferences* (pp. 2–8). New York: McGraw-Hill.

Greenberg, L., Andrea, G. D., & Lorence, D. (2004). Setting the public agenda for online health search: A white paper and action agenda. *Journal of Medical Internet Research, 6* (2), e8. Retrieved July 14, 2004, from http://www.jmir.org/2004/2/e18/index.htm.

Institute of Medicine of the National Academies (2003). *Health professions education: A bridge to quality.* Washington, DC: The National Academies Press.

Institute of Medicine of the National Academies (2004). *Patient safety: Achieving a new standard for care.* Washington, DC: The National Academies Press.

Masys, D. R., Brennan, P. F., Ozbolt, J. G., Corn, M., & Shortliffe, E. H. (2000). Are medical informatics and nursing informatics distinct disciplines? *Journal of American Medical Informatics Association, 7,* 304–312.

Moorhead, S., Johnson, M., & Maas, M. (Eds.) (2004). *Nursing outcomes classification* (NOC) 3rd ed. St. Louis: Mosby.

Murray, E., Lo, B., Pollack, L., Donelan, K.,Catania, J., Lee, K., Zapert, K., & Turner, R. (2003) The impact of health information on the Internet on health care and the physician-patient relationship: National U.S. survey among 1.050 U.S. physicians. A qualitative exploration. *Journal of Medical Internet Research, 5* (3), e17. Retrieved July 14, 2004, from http://www.jmir.org/2003/3/e17/index.htm.

National League for Nursing (2004). *Tri-council for nursing policy statement: Strategies to reverse the new nursing shortage.* Retrieved August 4, 2004, from http://www.nln.org/aboutnln/news_tricouncil2.htm.

Patt, M. R., Houston, T., K., Jenckes, M. W., Sands, D. Z., & Ford, D.E. (2003). Doctors who are using e-mail with their patients: A qualitative exploration. *Journal of Medical Internet Research, 5* (2), e9. Retrieved July 14, 2004, from http://www.jmir.org/2003/2/e9/index.htm.

Saba, V. K. (2001). Nursing informatics: Yesterday, today and tomorrow. *International Nursing Review, 48,* 177–187.

Saba, V. K. & McCormick, K. A. (Eds.) (2001). *Essentials of computers for nurses: Informatics in the next millennium.* New York: McGraw-Hill.

UK Health Informatics Society. What is Medical Informatics? Retrieved July 11, 2004, from http://www.bmis.org/what_is_mi.html.

Walji, M., Sagaram, S., Sagaram, D., Meric-Bernstam, F., Johnson, C., Mirza, N. Q., & Bernstam, E. V. (2004). Efficacy of quality criteria to identify potentially harmful information: A cross sectional survey of complementary and alternative medicine web sites. *Journal of Medical Internet Research, 6* (2), e9. Retrieved July 14, 2004, from http://www.jmir.org/2004/2/e21/index.htm.

Williams, M. D., Gish, K. W., Giuse, N. B., Sathe, N. A., & Carrell, D. L. (2001). The patient informatics consult service (PICS): An approach for a patient-centered service. *Bulletin of Medical Librarians Association, 89*(2), 185–193.

CHAPTER 10

Critical Thinking and Quality Improvement

The Institute of Medicine (IOM, 1990) defined quality as "the degree to which health services for individuals and populations increase the likelihood of desired health outcomes and are consistent with current professional knowledge" (p. 4). We believe they have retained this definition of quality over the years because it recognizes: 1) the impact healthcare has on quality of life for both patients and communities, 2) the probability of achieving better results, and 3) the reliability of those results stemming from sound information and critical thinking.

Based on the IOM definition, how would you rank healthcare quality today? Consider this question as it applies to your unit, your state, and nationally on a scale of 1–10. How high was your ranking? We propose that as a nation we are not close enough to "10" and therefore have a problem. Being generous, we'll label the problem "Inadequate Quality" as opposed to "Poor Quality."

This chapter examines the problem of inadequate quality healthcare while emphasizing the thinking we will need to solve the problem. Specifically we will explore: 1) the scope of the quality problem, 2) some history of efforts to achieve quality, 3) the relationship between quality and CT, and 4) the five IOM criteria for education and practice for applying quality improvement. We will demonstrate how CT is embedded in all of them.

SCOPE OF THE QUALITY PROBLEM

We probably all agree that the level of quality in healthcare would not receive a ranking of "10." In contemplating goals for remediation, we need to reflect on whether reaching "10" would be possible. Attempting to achieve perfection in complex systems is not only unrealistic, it may actually make matters worse. Attempts at perfection have a tendency to increase the level of system complexity, which in turn potentially leads to more system failures (Agency for Healthcare Research and Quality, 1999).

Recognizing the inadequate quality of healthcare in this country and that achieving perfection is unrealistic, we can search for data to define the scope of the problem using the CT dimensions of *inquisitiveness, information seeking,* and *analysis. Inquisitiveness* drives us to explore, find out what is working, what is not, and why. *Information seeking* enables us to gather useful data, and *analysis* allows us to examine the parts of the problem in manageable segments so we can thoroughly study the problem before looking for solutions. As you will see, discovering those solutions will require additional CT dimensions.

The Institute of Medicine (IOM) was one of the first healthcare groups to ask questions about quality. In the early 1990s the IOM raised awareness of the over-use, misuse, and under-use of healthcare services in the U.S.A. At that point the IOM recommended switching to computer-based patient records as a way of monitoring healthcare issues. ("Informatics" enters the picture.) Computerized data provided the means to find out how serious the problem with quality was (IOM, 2004a).

In 2000 the IOM issued *To Err is Human: Building a Safer Health System*, and in 2001, *Crossing the Quality Chasm: A New Health System for the 21st Century*. Both of these reports revealed growing concerns about quality in health-care. The data from the US healthcare system revealed that on a yearly basis:

- 7% of patients suffer a medication error
- Every patient admitted to an ICU suffers an adverse event
- 44,000 to 98,000 deaths [result from errors]
- $50 billion in total costs [result from errors] (Pronovost, 2004)

Although these data are specific to the US system, Pronovost noted similar results in the United Kingdom and Australia.

Data patterns reflected "near misses" and "adverse events." Near misses were defined as "acts of omission or commission that could have harmed the patient but did not cause harm as a result of chance, prevention or mitigation" (IOM, 2004a, p. 227). An adverse event was "an event that results in unintended harm to the patient by an act of commission or omission rather than by the underlying disease or condition of the patient" (IOM, 2004a, p. 201).

The most severe adverse event, "sentinel event," was identified by the Joint Commission on the Accreditation of Healthcare Organizations (JCAHO) as "an unexpected occurrence involving death or serious physical—including loss of limb or function—or psychological injury, or the risk thereof. 'Risk there of' means that, although no harm occurred this time, any recurrence would carry a significant chance of a serious adverse outcome" ("Facts about Patient Safety" n.d.).

JCAHO produces a monthly newsletter that reports on sentinel events. The July 2004 report indicated 2,667 patients had been affected by sentinel events since JCAHO began to collect data in January 1995. Seventy-five percent of those events resulted in death, with the top five causes being: patient suicide, operative and post operative complications, wrong site surgery, and medica-tion error ("This Month at the Joint Commission" July 15, 2004).

JCAHO also publishes a *Sentinel Event ALERT*, which includes a root cause analysis of one problem area at a time. The July 21, 2004 report updated the number of perinatal deaths to 61 and permanent disabilities to 10 for a total of 71 sentinel events in the perinatal category. The "root cause" of these events was attributed to the organizational culture that hindered effective communication and teamwork ("Sentinel Event ALERT" July 21, 2004).

The 2004 IOM report, *Keeping Patients Safe: Transforming the Work Environment of Nurses,* added an additional dimension to the problem with quality in reference to the 44,000 to 98,000 deaths from errors: "This alarming number, which reflects only deaths occurring in hospital settings, . . . does not reflect the many patients who survive, but sustain serious injuries" (2004b, p. 1). Thus, most "adverse events" and all "near misses" are not addressed in this data.

The IOM also noted that the 98,000 figure for deaths from errors far exceeded deaths from other causes, including motor vehicle accidents, breast cancer, or AIDS. These are some serious numbers. Our attention to quality and the thinking required to achieve it can no longer be just words in a mission statement or an esoteric classroom discussion.

On our path to a solution, the next logical question is, "How did this happen?" Have we not been paying attention to quality over the years? We need some historical perspective here to see how efforts to achieve quality in healthcare have evolved. It may be time for some new thinking considering all the data showing how healthcare has become increasingly risky.

BRIEF HISTORY OF QUALITY IMPROVEMENT

Besides looking at early efforts to improve quality in healthcare, this section identifies the problems inherent in past and present solutions. It also identifies some of the public and private organizations that find the current situation in healthcare unacceptable.

The terminology describing early efforts to achieve quality was "quality assurance." Applications of quality assurance measures first were applied to business and industry. They focused on finding mistakes *after* they occurred (for example, discovering problems with an automobile after it had been fully assembled). The result of that approach was to identify the person or point in the assembly operation responsible for the mistakes/errors. Quality assurance focused on parts of the system, but not the whole system itself (Shortell, Bennett, & Byck, 1998).

Donabedian, considered to be the founder of healthcare quality assurance, began his work in the 1960s. His healthcare model was a synthesis of business models of quality assurance and public health quality needs. Donabedian (2003) addressed structure, process, and outcomes as components of quality assessment in healthcare. Although his language implied a whole systems approach, that did not pan out in reality because healthcare providers had difficulty conceptualizing strategies to deal with whole systems.

A shift in thinking and terminology that enhanced a system focus has evolved over the last few decades. "Quality assurance" projects converted to "continuous quality improvement" (CQI) when the need to deal with the whole system could no longer be ignored. New goals included preventing errors before they occurred and identifying problems within the system, or subsystem, rather than blaming the individual (Shortell, Bennett, & Byck, 1998).

CQI also began in the business and industry sectors prior to being introduced into healthcare in the late 1980s. By the early 1990s, 69% of U.S. hospitals began implementing some form of CQI. Early CQI efforts in healthcare focused primarily on structural issues such as administrative activities dealing with scheduling, billing procedures, and patient appointments. Not until the late 1990s did CQI projects begin to examine clinical process issues such as medication errors (Shortell et al., 1998).

Problems with Past and Present Approaches

As mentioned above, the "quality assurance" approach did not work well in healthcare, as it: 1) focused on identifying problems after they occurred, and 2) was not implemented as a systems approach. Although CQI has been widely embraced for years as a strategy for quality improvement, it has two fundamental problems as well. First, the focus of CQI was too narrow because it concentrated primarily on structure and/or processes and not on outcomes or whole systems. Second, CQI had and still has limited research to support its effectiveness (Shortell et al., 1998; Alemi, 1999).

Too Narrow a Focus

Looking at structure and/or process alone has not led to quality outcomes. A logical move is to include outcomes in evaluation plans. The question then becomes one of defining those outcomes: "What are quality outcomes in healthcare?"

Healthcare and education are increasingly being expected to demonstrate a certain kind of outcome these days. We are no longer looking for process outcomes that answer questions such as, "were the correct medications given?" Instead, we seek outcomes that measure changes in the patient or the student as a result of what we did "to them." The terminology "value added results" has become synonymous with this revised approach to outcomes, implying an end product, or a result of some process that is better at the exit point than at the entry point. To assess "value added results"/outcomes related to quality healthcare, we need to ask different questions than the ones we have been asking, such as: "How are patients who leave the hospital after treatment different from when they entered the hospital?" Similar quality outcome questions are being asked in higher education, such as: "How are university graduates different than they were when they were admitted four years earlier?"

Whether we are measuring quality healthcare or quality education we must move beyond a narrow focus on structure and process to address issues of results, that is, quality outcomes. *And* we have to tackle quality in the broadest sense, for the whole system and not just the parts. That will take more thinking. Surprise! Surprise! ☺

A broader focus on quality outcomes in healthcare requires at least *perseverance, discriminating*, and *contextual perspective. Perseverance* drives our search for the best ways to describe outcomes (for example, patient safety vs. quality care). *Discriminating* helps us avoid confusing process (giving the correct medication) with patient results/outcomes (how the patient reacted to the medication), and *discriminating* helps to judge the quality of the outcomes: good, better, and best outcomes. *Contextual perspective* helps us see the big picture; i.e., the relationships among parts in the system and to the whole system with all its complexity.

Limited Research Support for CQI

There is little evidence that CQI really works. The research that is cited is generally positive, but because so few unsuccessful projects have reached publication we cannot use our *analysis* and *logical reasoning* to make valid comparisons among them. The few randomized studies that have reached publication show no relationship between CQI activities and clinical outcomes or improved clinical performance (Shortell et al., 1998; Alemi, 1999). Without research evidence, it is difficult to support or advocate for the ongoing use of CQI in healthcare.

IOM (2003) summarized the problems with past and present quality improvement movements, noting the obstacles as: 1) lack of adequate information infrastructures, 2) unprepared leadership, and 3) sparse well-designed research studies providing evidence of improved patient outcomes in healthcare as a result of CQI projects.

Who Is Concerned About Quality in Healthcare?

The desire to achieve quality is gaining momentum in spite of the obstacles and gaps in research. Problems of quality care are increasing with regularity. Organizations concerned with quality are mushrooming; they all use language that implies CT, such as, ". . . in studying an *intuitively* plausible 'risk factor' for errors, such as 'fatigue,' *analyses* of errors commonly reveal the presence of fatigued providers . . ." [we added the italics for emphasis on the thinking language] (AHRQ, 1999,

---

Box 10.1

Groups and Organizations Addressing Quality in Healthcare

Institute of Medicine (IOM): www.iom.edu/

Agency for Healthcare Research and Quality (AHRQ): www.ahrq.gov

National Committee for Quality Assurance (NCQA): www.ncqu.org

Joint Commission on Accreditation of Healthcare Organizations (JCAHO): www.jcaho.org

National Quality Forum (NQF): www.qualityforum.org

The Leapfrog Group for Patient Safety: www.leapfrog.org

IPRO Quality Improvement Organization: www.ipro.org

Center for Patient Safety: www.asph.org/patient-safety/

Talking Quality.gov: www.talkingquality.gov/default.html

---

p. 3). Such organizations study and advocate for accurate information, emphasizing the need for collaborative thinking and discussion to find creative solutions.

Box 10.1 identifies a random selection of the many public and private groups and organizations concerned with quality in healthcare. The *Health: Public Health and Safety: Patient Safety* website listed below includes another 55 organizations that can be accessed to receive updated information about quality and safety, http://dmox.org/Health/Public_Health_and_Safety/Patient_Safety/.

With all this growing concern to improve quality in healthcare, how can we make sure we do not end up going in circles using past approaches? The answers include: 1) looking more closely at the relationship between quality and thinking, and 2) re-thinking quality improvement.

RELATIONSHIP BETWEEN QUALITY AND CT

Quality in healthcare is an outcome of good thinking, or should we say great thinking! Figure 10.1 returns to the medallion symbol first used in Chapter 5 to represent "applying quality improvement." We selected this symbol because it generally represents a mark of excellence or an award for great work.

This more detailed illustration of the medallion identifies three standards of quality: safe, effective, and efficient care. Surrounding those three standards is a ring representing interdisciplinary team thinking and, beyond that ring, are the 17 dimensions of CT. The medallion ribbons represent the "desired health outcomes" of the IOM definition of quality cited earlier in this chapter.

The whole represents the Medallion of Quality Healthcare Through Critical Thinking. Thinking starts with each individual provider, but then joins the

Figure 10.1   Medallion of Quality Healthcare Through Critical Thinking

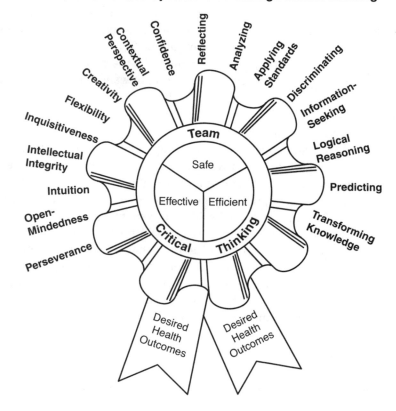

thinking of others, including the patient. For the remainder of this chapter we will use CT to represent both individual and interdisciplinary thinking. It is this collaborative thinking that ultimately changes rankings of quality from good to better to best.

RE-THINKING QUALITY IMPROVEMENT

Now let's return to the problem of inadequate quality in healthcare. We know what does not work—quality assurance and CQI. Our re-thinking starts with one "Don't" and two "Dos." We *don't* want to revert to using old solutions under new names. We *do* want to acknowledge the complexity of the healthcare system, and we *do* want to expand our thinking to match these new levels of complexity. We then need to apply that new level of thinking to some specific quality criteria.

The "Don't"

One of the common errors in all problem solving is re-naming something and thinking it is a new solution. Except for the re-naming, Albert Einstein referred to this recycling of solutions by saying, "Doing the same thing over and over again and expecting different results: [is the definition of] Insanity" ("Famous quotes, Einstein quotes," n.d.) We do not want to go down that path!

The First "Do"

We do want to acknowledge the complexity of healthcare and its demands for new levels of thinking and problem solving. Healthcare systems have moved well beyond complicated and into the realm of complex. Complex systems are not like machines; they are more like conscious entities (Wheatley, 1994) or living organisms. As such, healthcare systems are constantly adaptive (Plsek, 2003). In other words, people, responsibilities, and workloads do not stay in their nice little boxes on organizational charts. Structure, process, and patterns of relationships are dynamic and constantly changing. These characteristics must be actively addressed when looking for solutions for inadequate quality in healthcare. Chapter 11 will discuss in more detail this very important issue of complexity and its impact on change.

The Second "Do"

Thinking in systems is another level of thinking. All of the systems thinking strategies we discussed in Chapter 7 play a part. Another observation from Einstein hits the nail on the head regarding the need for change in thinking: "The significant problems we face cannot be solved at the same level of thinking we were at when we created them" ("Famous quotes, Einstein quotes," n.d.).

We're not sure which parts of thinking "created" the problems of quality in healthcare, but we are certain it will take all 17 CT dimensions to deal with their current level of complexity.

Applying a New Level of Thinking

Now, for some serious "new level" thinking about quality improvement. Notice we said *new level*. We will still need the basic 17 dimensions of CT, but we need to use more of them, more often, and involve the thinking of more people. We'll start with some good old fashioned *analysis* to see the pieces. Here is a capsule version of what we know:

#1 Quality is an outcome deemed important in healthcare.

#2 Quality is declining as evident by the growing numbers of errors in healthcare leading to both serious injury or death.

#3 Both consumers and providers are becoming very alarmed.

#4 CQI has no solid research to support its effectiveness in producing quality patient outcomes.

The next steps, *logical reasoning* and *inquisitiveness*, lead to a major question: "Just what is quality?" There is the very broad IOM definition cited at the beginning of this chapter. The IOM definition gives us the idea but not the specifics; it is too nebulous to be useful in identifying what specifically needs to be done. We have to do some *information seeking, transforming knowledge*, and *applying standards* to: 1) clarify what we mean by quality, 2) design strategies to achieve quality, and 3) figure out if we achieved it. The bottom line is we need more specific criteria to identify quality.

Luckily the IOM (2003) expanded its definition by establishing five criteria for the educational changes necessary to improved quality in healthcare. As you read these five criteria, in Box 10.2 below, think about what is needed to change healthcare practice, education, *and* thinking patterns to move in those directions. Our new level of thinking requires clinicians and educators to engage as many of the 17 CT dimensions as possible and as often as possible.

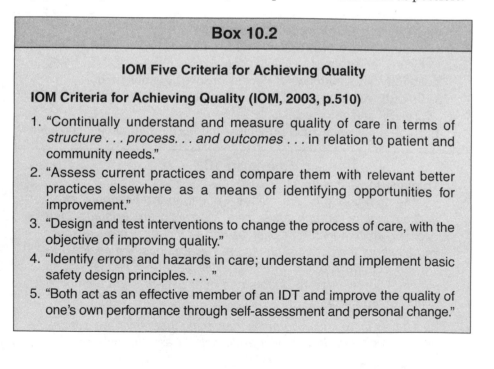

Box 10.2

IOM Five Criteria for Achieving Quality

IOM Criteria for Achieving Quality (IOM, 2003, p.510)

1. "Continually understand and measure quality of care in terms of *structure . . . process. . . and outcomes . . .* in relation to patient and community needs."
2. "Assess current practices and compare them with relevant better practices elsewhere as a means of identifying opportunities for improvement."
3. "Design and test interventions to change the process of care, with the objective of improving quality."
4. "Identify errors and hazards in care; understand and implement basic safety design principles. . . . "
5. "Both act as an effective member of an IDT and improve the quality of one's own performance through self-assessment and personal change."

Although all 17 CT dimensions are necessary to achieve the five IOM criteria, only some will be used in our examples for the sake of time and also to allow you to discover the others. Each criterion and its necessary CT will be discussed separately for the remainder of the chapter.

IOM CRITERION #1

> **#1** Continually understand and measure quality of care in terms of "structure," or the inputs into the system, such as patients, staff, and environments; "process," or the interactions between clinicians and patients; and "outcomes," or evidence about changes in patients' health status in relation to patient and community needs (IOM, 2003, p. 59).

This criterion actually returns to the quality assurance concepts of structure, process, and outcomes discussed by Donabedian in the 1960s. Structure, process, and outcomes are valuable concepts in healthcare, but are more valuable when all three are looked at as a whole. Remember the saying, "The whole is greater than the sum of its parts"? Basically this means we have to recognize the whole as its own conscious entity in addition to the contributions of its parts.

To illustrate how these three concepts work together as a system, and the thinking involved, complete TACTICS 10.1, which uses Scenario 10.1.

TACTICS 10.1 Thinking for Criterion #1

1. Read Scenario 10.1. Notice we have inserted some of the CT used by the nurses.
2. Identify any additional CT dimensions we have not cited.
3. Identify the aspects of this situation that represent structure, process, and outcomes.
4. Think about some other possible solutions the staff did not consider.

Scenario 10.1

Thinking for Criterion #1

The community health nurses working in the well-baby clinic noticed that fewer and fewer new mothers were bringing their babies in for immunizations over the last six months. They were concerned about the potential for increasing incidence of measles during the coming months when measles generally peaks among infants. They wanted to understand both patient and community needs. (Predicting)

They want to find out what is happening that may have precipitated this change in behavior and begin to ask the mothers that *come if they have any ideas. They also consult the CDC website to see if this is a national or regional occurrence or unique to their clinic. They consult pediatrician offices as well. **(Information seeking)***

*The mothers who visit the clinic have no idea what the problem could be; they are very pleased with the service they receive. The CDC website has no indication that this is a widespread problem; local pediatrician offices have not experienced the problem either. The nurses, however, are not about to give up. They meet with the other clinic staff and try to brainstorm ideas. Are they doing something to discourage the return of certain patients? Are they missing some culturally sensitive information considering they serve a population of rural migrant workers? Maybe the parents have been listening to the news reports about mercury in the immunizations causing autism and are afraid of immunizing their children. **(Perseverance, open-mindedness, intellectual integrity)***

The nurses decide to try to contact the new mothers directly to ask them what is happening. Because few have phones, they make several home visits and ask about the missed appointments. They get only vague excuses about not having time or forgetting.

*While driving to a final home visit, the nurse begins to think about one forgotten piece of the whole process of immunizations—access to service. She notices that all of the bus stops that used to be in this part of the county are no longer there. When she arrives at the home she asks the mother about the missed appointments, gets the same vague answer, and then asks about the missing bus stops. **(Contextual perspective)***

*With some encouragement the mother admits that she does not have enough money for a taxi to bring her daughter to the clinic for her immunizations. The nurse compares the dates of the decline in immunization appointments with the date the busses stopped servicing some areas of the county and found a match. She and the rest of the clinic team know that declining immunizations puts the children as well as the community at risk. They combine their thinking and discuss how to approach this situation using the structure, process, outcomes framework recommended by the IOM. **(Analysis, logical reasoning)***

Discussion

What other CT dimensions did you identify? What did you see as structure, process, and outcomes? Initially the staff thought the lack of culturally sensitive interventions for immunizations might be a process problem. It turned out to be a structural problem—transportation. What started as an observation by an inquisitive nurse (declining immunization appointments in a well-baby clinic) became a broader system issue that required CT as the nurses and others examined the structure, process, and outcomes.

The thinking about "structure" included perspectives from the parents of the under-immunized children, transportation authorities who make bus routes, city officials who provide tax money to the transportation authority, and volunteer agencies that provide free transportation. Thinking about "process" included collaboration with all parties to examine causes as well as solutions—for example, considering if the staff were culturally sensitive to this population's needs. Thinking about outcomes ultimately focused on the rates of immunization and ultimately led to an increase in quality of health of the children and the community.

If the staff in the clinic had gone even further in their thinking, they would have *reflected* on the overall system and how immunization outcomes could be more assured. They might identify ways to use what they learned to deal with other current and future problems. They may have begun to think about how to create a system of mobile satellite clinics providing access to the full range of healthcare services for families in outlying areas. And they might have thought about how to seek grant money to fund the project.

IOM CRITERIA #2 AND #3

#2 Assess current practices and compare them with relevant better practices elsewhere as a means of identifying opportunities for improvement.

#3 Design and test interventions to change the process of care with the objective of improving quality (IOM, 2003, p. 59).

These two criteria are being discussed together because they both deal with evidence-based practice (EBP). Refer to Chapter 8 for details on EBP. Criterion #2 implies the use of evidence-based guidelines that would be the "relevant better practices" as comparisons to current practice. Comparisons require *information seeking* to locate the best practice guidelines and *applying standards* to select the best fit.

Criterion #3 then pushes for implementation of best practice and testing how the change in practice makes things better. We discussed the CT required for EBP in detail in Chapter 8. As a quick refresher, consider *flexibility, creativity, transforming knowledge,* and *contextual perspective. Flexibility* helps clinicians adjust practices as better evidence emerges. *Creativity* is particularly necessary for finding ways to implement evidence-based guidelines. *Trans-*

forming knowledge is used to find evidence and translate it into practice. And *contextual perspective* helps customize best practices to the individual patient.

Criteria #2 and #3 and the incorporation of EBP ultimately lead to safe, effective, and efficient care. The IOM (2000) addressed six attributes for quality health care systems: "(1) safe, (2) effective, (3) patient centered, (4) timely, (5) efficient, and (6) equitable." (pp. 41–42). Of those six, effective and efficient/timely care fit well with criteria #2 and #3 and are discussed below. Patient-centered care was discussed in Chapter 6. Equitable care has not been addressed in this book, but is a serious concern today and certainly will be so tomorrow. Safe care is discussed with IOM Criterion #4.

Effective Care

Effective care refers to providing the right type and amount of care to specifically address the problem at hand. The right type of care should be what is recommended by solid evidence. We use CT, specifically *logical reasoning*, to accurately match data and conclusions drawn from those data sets with interventions.

Matching the data with conclusions, matching the right provider to patient needs, and matching appropriate tests and procedures to patient conditions are essential aspects of effective care. This can be a delicate balancing act. Providers need to avoid overdoing things, such as ordering unnecessary tests or procedures. Not everyone with neck pain needs an MRI or CAT scan. Antibiotics are not proper treatment for viral infections. Patients with back pain do not necessarily need orthopedic surgery; many will do much better with treatment from a physical therapist specializing in back pain.

Over-use is wasteful and under-use can lead to errors and death. For example, for a patient who complains of headaches and is diagnosed and treated for migraines but has a brain tumor, care is not effective. The best CT along with the best evidence make the difference between effective quality and ineffective quality healthcare.

Effectiveness has implications for CT in teaching as well, whether it is in the academic classroom or practice setting. Scenario 10.2 illustrates the problems that ensue when quality thinking impacts teaching and quality care.

Scenario 10.2
Earl's Staff Development Teaching Effectiveness
Earl is a staff-development instructor for a 30-bed step-down unit in an urban hospital. It is time to do his annual in-service on care of central lines to meet JCAHO standards. He has done this

several times over the last couple years and pulls out his file with lecture notes, grabs the video off the shelf, runs to make copies of the quiz he designed when he first prepared the material, and heads off to the conference room.

During his presentation two nurses seem to be napping, but they scored fine on the quiz so he decides not to say anything. The one new staff member, Jill, however, did not score well. He decides he'd better meet with her and review some of the material. When he talks with Jill, she tells him she learned to do central line dressings differently in school and that's why she answered the way she did. Earl says he will check that out.

Later that week at the weekly staff meeting the new unit manager shares some data she has been collecting on quality and notices the increasing frequency of infections for patients having central lines on this unit.

Earl looks surprised and says, "I don't know how that can be. I've been doing in-services on central lines consistently for the last few years and everyone attends and passes the post quiz. I hope we aren't getting another strain of staph on the unit."

TACTICS 10.2 Thinking and Effectiveness

After reading Scenario 10.2, identify the CT skills and habits of the mind that were not used.

Discussion

The obvious missing CT dimensions are these:

- No *information seeking* on Earl's part to update his information. (He clearly did not read Chapter 8 of this book!)
- No *reflection* on Earl's part to consider examining his information, teaching style, or measurement instrument before or after his teaching.
- No evidence of *inquisitiveness* to find out about changes in central line care since he first prepared his teaching material, and to ask why Jill has different information.
- No *intellectual integrity* on Earl's part to explore the possibility that he might not be teaching accurate information.

One of the significant areas of improvement would be for Earl to use EBP. Earl could have done a literature review or gone to the Internet (the CDC would have been a good place to start) to look up the latest practice guidelines for central lines. This would have provided him with a better match for the problem, central line care and the proper interventions, thus promoting effective care as opposed to outdated practice. This behavior requires using at least the CT dimensions listed above, plus most other dimensions. Give yourself some stars for additional ones we did not list, and if you see Earl, tell him about evidence-based practice.

Efficient Care

Criteria #2 and #3 also expect efficient care. "Efficiency . . . calls for conducting production activities in as cost-effective and time-efficient manner as possible" (IOM, 2004b, p. 114). Again, balance is important. Excessive cost-cutting measures without attention to quality frequently lead to decreased staffing, less equipment, and fewer opportunities for catching errors. An example of useful efficiency measures would be to *analyze* a procedure that has 50 steps, look at all its parts, and see how it could be simplified (by using *logical reasoning*) to determine what could be safely eliminated. If that procedure could be reduced to 35 steps without sacrificing safety, then time, money, and energy would be saved.

Scenario 10.3 below illustrates the problems with efficiency in a Breast Care Clinic.

Scenario 10.3
Making Care More Efficient for Allison

Allison experienced a problem with the length of time it took to get her annual mammogram. When she scheduled her appointment she was told to plan to be there as long as two hours. This seemed long, but at least she was prepared for that and took papers to grade. The appointment was scheduled for 11:00. She arrived at 10:45. She was called in from the first waiting room to undress and put on a "house-coat" type gown for the exam at 11:30. After changing she waited another 20 minutes in the inner waiting room with several other women before being escorted to an examination room for her breast exam at 11:50 then back to the inner waiting room. The actual mammogram was done in yet another room at 12:30. After the mammogram she went back to the inner waiting room and waited, and waited, and waited. After the doctor was free to review the films, she was told things were fine and she should come back in a year. By then it was 2:00 in the afternoon. Allison was one of six women who spent up to 4 hours waiting that day.

Allison was very upset and spoke with the clinic manager. She was told it took that long because the doctor wanted to talk to everyone personally even if the results were normal. Not satisfied with that answer, Allison wrote a letter reiterating her concern and adding a suggestion that if they planned to keep patients that long they should at least feed them.

Allison put off her next mammogram for three years. Due to the difficulty in finding another provider she finally went back to the clinic and was pleasantly surprised to find she was in and out in less than two hours. She wasn't involved in the change, but decided her letter may have helped either start it or add fuel to the fire. She was pleased she had the confidence *to speak up.*

TACTICS 10.3 Thinking and Efficiency

1. After reading Scenario 10.3 identify how CT affected efficiency.
2. How would you describe the efficiency of Allison's care?
3. Identify what thinking skills and habits of the mind were used to make the care more efficient for Allison.

Discussion

How do you think Allison felt about the efficiency of this process? For those of you who have had a mammogram, you know it is not the most comfortable procedure in the world; having it take over four hours, when the appointment was planned for two hours, may very likely discourage regular examinations in the future. The decreased efficiency led to decreased effectiveness.

So what thinking is needed here? Allison did some on her own, using her *confidence*, but what might the office team have done to make this change in efficiency? *Analysis* helps through examining parts of a system that are not working the way they should—those that put up roadblocks to quality care delivery. *Flexibility* helps to make changes. *Open-mindedness* helps the staff to listen to patient concerns.

In the Breast Care Clinic, the office team was apparently concerned enough about patient-centered care (it's unlikely Allison was the only one who complained) and coming up with ways to streamline the process. By becoming more efficient, they increased the chances that patients would return for their routine visits and thus improved quality outcomes—early detection of breast cancer.

IOM CRITERION #4

#4 Identify errors and hazards in care; understand and implement basic safety design principles, such as standardization and simplification and human factors training (IOM, 2003, p. 59).

Criterion #4 is aimed at safe care. Safety is the "gold standard" for quality these days. Safety is also something that is very amenable to thinking. *Analysis, logical reasoning, inquisitiveness, predicting,* and *intellectual integrity* are only five of the 17 CT dimensions necessary to prevent errors and hazards. Because there is a lot of material in this section, we have provided a roadmap to help you stay on track.

We start with a TACTICS to examine a safety issue in healthcare. From there we: 1) discuss errors and hazards that hinder safety and how they are categorized, 2) explore how the current organizational culture influences error identification, and 3) identify solutions for better safety. TACTICS 10.4 and the accompanying scenario were selected to demonstrate the relationship between safety and error identification.

TACTICS 10.4 CT for Assessing Safety

1. Read Scenario 10.4.
2. Find the dimensions of thinking that are used *and* those that are missing.
3. Determine what kind of errors, if any, are present in this situation.

Scenario 10.4

Mr. Davis

Mr. Davis is being discharged today and has a list of medications he needs to take at home. He has been taking Celexa during his hospital stay. His nurse, Betty, who is staffing five patients today because someone called in sick, is in a rush to give blood and doesn't notice the order for Celebrex instead of Celexa. She asks Sara, who just came on, to help out and finish the discharge teaching for Mr. Davis.

Sara is new to this unit; she examines the discharge meds before going in to teach Mr. Davis. She doesn't recognize the name of one drug on the list, Celebrex, but notices from the chart that it looks like what Mr. Davis has been taking. Sara looks for the drug book to check it out, but can't find it. She sees Mr. Davis' doctor rushing off the unit and doesn't want to bother him. She calls the pharmacy, but the line is busy and just then Mrs. Davis arrives at the nurses' station.

Mrs. Davis says she has the dog in the car and it's hot outside; she has Mr. Davis all set in the wheelchair and is ready to go.

Sara escorts Mr. Davis to the hospital entrance, reminding him to get his prescriptions filled as soon as possible and to call if he has any questions. Mr. Davis goes home with a prescription for Celebrex instead of Celexa.

Discussion

What do you think is the likelihood of this happening? We hope it is not common, but considering the national and international nursing shortage, its potential is rising. Did you find some use of CT dimensions? We came up with these missing CT dimensions. Compare our list with yours and, for all additional dimensions you thought of, give yourself an extra star, or if you're lucky enough to be slim, have chocolate! If you're not so slim, have the chocolate anyway, but take a break from reading and go for a walk.

Missing Thinking

Insufficient *discrimination* of the different medications by Betty and Sara.

Insufficient *applying standards* relative to medication administration by Sara.

Beginning *perseverance* but not enough by Sara in identifying the medication discrepancy.

No *confidence* in her reasoning as Sara does not pursue her concerns.

As part of our CT we would look to the system for ways to protect Mr. Davis and other patients from taking the wrong medication. JCAHO recommended attention to what they refer to as "high alert medications," that is, medications with similar names, similar packaging, not commonly used, or commonly used that trigger allergic reactions. Attention also should be given to ones that require close monitoring or testing (for example, lithium, warfarin, digoxin, and theophylline) (as cited in Benner, 2001). Mr. Davis would have benefited from his nurses' CT and attention to medications with similar names.

Also, think about who needs to participate in team thinking about how to decrease medication errors. How could those participants create system strategies to alert staff to commonly misread medication names? What should they think about besides assigning blame to individuals? Hold that thought; we'll talk more about a culture of safety shortly.

Errors and Hazards

Safe care is achieved by employing EBP; error and hazard identification is enhanced by informatics. Healthcare is so complex that it is foolish to think "things won't go wrong." Once we accept that, we can constructively look for errors and hazards and realistically seek to improve safety for patients.

Again we need to examine the concepts. What are the errors and hazards? How do we recognize them? In general, "error" can mean collecting insufficient data, making the wrong diagnoses, giving the wrong medications and/or providing the wrong treatments by the wrong providers. All these wrongs can result in a continuum of unacceptable outcomes, from delays in care to death, with pain and suffering along the way. Those "wrongs" are officially labeled "adverse events" and "near misses."

Adverse Events and Near Misses

We defined "adverse events" and "near misses" at the beginning of this chapter, but we'll repeat them here to refresh your memory as we elaborate on the concepts. An "adverse event" is "an event that results in unintended harm to the patient by an act of commission or omission rather than by the underlying disease or condition of the patient" (IOM, 2004a, p. 201).

These events (errors) are frequently attributed to the poor design, communication patterns, and organization of the healthcare delivery system, not individuals. Such errors generally lead to incident reports and, if the errors lead to death or permanent injury, a sentinel event report. Nurses and others need "not only the knowledge to recognize an error, but also the confidence and communication skills to address the issue with appropriate personnel" (Henneman & Gawlinski, 2004, p. 200). That requires both *confidence* (in reasoning) and *intellectual integrity*.

"Near misses" are defined as "acts of omission or commission that could have harmed the patient but did not cause harm as a result of chance, prevention or mitigation" (IOM, 2004a, p. 227). Near misses occur frequently, as much as 100 times more frequently than "adverse events." Depending on the organizational culture, "near miss" data may or may not be reported. *Perseverance* is important in paying attention to patterns and consistently collecting data that are needed to document those patterns and make changes.

Eindhover Model of Errors

Errors can be examined from other perspectives as well. The Eindhover Model is cited by IOM (2004a) as one way to incorporate "near misses" and "adverse events" into the broader perspective of technical, human, and organizational failures. The model is based on the premise that safety mechanisms can be implemented to prevent errors (Henneman & Gawlinski, 2004). Using the term "failure" from the Eindhoven Model can have negative connotations, but the value of the model lies in examining errors from the perspective of a technical, human, and organizational framework. Analyzing these parts of the complex healthcare system are only useful, however, if they are ultimately examined together as a whole.

Technical failures occur in computer systems, hardware or software, and malfunctioning equipment. This is a growing problem as equipment ages and funding shrinks.

The second type of failure in the Eindhoven model, human failure, has actually been shown to be less responsible than system errors for adverse events (Gloe, 1998; IOM, 2001). Yet human failures cannot be ignored. The IOM (2004b) noted that even though only about 10% of unsafe acts are due to individuals, ignoring that 10% would be very dangerous.

Leape identified "cognitive mechanisms" and "cognitive processes" as two thinking aspects of human error (Leape, 1994). Cognitive mechanisms are essential habitual behaviors used over and over to carry out some task. They require little attention, but can be derailed by interruptions, fatigue, time pressures, and emotions such as fear, anxiety, and boredom. It is hard to imagine spending a day caring for patients without interruptions and time pressures interfering with thinking.

Cognitive processes, on the other hand, require higher levels of thinking, focused attention, knowledge, and critical decision making. When cognitive processes are not up to par, decisions are hindered by misinterpretation of data, insufficient knowledge or experience, overdependence on cognitive mechanisms, and not basing actions on the most current knowledge (Affonso & Doran, 2002). Dysfunctions in cognitive mechanisms and/or cognitive processes can lead to inaccurate decisions and potentially lethal safety errors.

Organizational failure, the third source of errors, generally refers to problems with the structures and processes employed to run an organization—all the strategic plans, policies, procedures, and protocols. Organizations can promote or impede safety efforts as a function of their cultural norms.

Organizational Culture Influences on Error Identification

Organizations are not inanimate objects; they are groups of people who relate, interact, think, and work together for many hours each day. Organizations, therefore, have all of the characteristics of any group of people, including a culture. Cultures have values, beliefs, and attitudes that influence behaviors such as identifying errors.

Westrum and Gleason (2003) examined the current healthcare culture and found several values, beliefs, and attitudes that actually promote errors. They cited "finding someone to blame" as a predominant factor hindering the recognition of errors. Other factors suppressing problems included "spinning" a more acceptable version of a problem, and looking for a quick fix.

All these factors stifle cognitive inquiry and quality in healthcare organizations. Westrum and Gleason went on to emphasize the lack of opportunities to think together as one of the primary hindrances for identification of potential and actual errors in healthcare cultures. (That's a cue to appreciate interdisciplinary teams. See Chapter 7!)

Although healthcare cultures vary, historically all have had two traditional values and beliefs: 1) avoiding all errors is possible, and 2) finding the one or more persons who are to blame for an error (IOM, 2004b). We must transform our thinking about the myth that we can avoid all errors because it is counterproductive to developing a new culture of safety. Old beliefs and attitudes about perfection and avoiding errors severely limit our ability to collect accurate data for research and decisions on system changes.

We must also move beyond blaming individuals. According to Benner (2001), a culture of blame and shame actually discourages the reporting of errors for fear of punishment and being singled out for responsibility. Organizational cultures that retain values of blaming and pretending all errors can be avoided ultimately have a much more difficult job of improving quality (Henneman & Gawlinski ((2004).

Safety Solutions

Solutions for better safety are essential to the ultimate goal of quality improvement. This section focuses on the CT needed to: 1) move to a culture of safety, 2) devise/find and implement processes for collection and monitoring errors in healthcare, and 3) develop safety goals.

Culture of Safety

Healthcare providers must be open and attentive to finding their errors, errors of others, and errors in the system, and not be overtly or covertly punished in the process. If the current culture hinders that openness and attentiveness, the obvious solution is to change the culture. The question is, change it to what?

Benner (2001) had two suggestions for changing the healthcare culture to a focus on safety. One is to accept the fact that "practice is broader and more flexible than the science and technology that support practice" (p. 283). Clinicians who accept that and educators who teach that will be promoting a culture of safety, one that acknowledges the need for *flexibility* and *contextual perspective* in the CT of providers. Benner's second suggestion was to focus on self-improvement, which requires *reflection*. Both self *reflection* and *reflection* on the organizational system are essential to changing a culture. We'll discuss this issue of *reflection* in more detail with criterion #5.

Affonso and Doran (2002) also address solutions for changing the healthcare culture. Their version calls for revolutionary thinking to develop a science of safety by encouraging *creative* thinking. Their conceptual framework focuses on patient safety through research, education, and practice by creating conditions for critical thinking, ethical practice, and opportunities for learning.

The IOM (2004b) *Keeping Patients Safe: Transforming the Work Environment of Nurses* confirms the need for more opportunities for thinking to sustain a culture of safety. An entire chapter (Creating and Sustaining a Culture of Safety) of that report addressed issues of: 1) empowering employees with decision-making rights, 2) encouraging staff to question orders with *confidence*, 3) using *creativity* to think of ways to improve procedures, 4) developing their *prediction* abilities to anticipate adverse events, and 5) being able to use *discrimination* abilities to make decisions and select the best practice interventions. The italics are ours; by now you know why we added them.

CT is also essential for transformational leadership and evidence-based management. The IOM (2004b) emphasized the need for top management to "provide time for thinking, learning and training . . . employees must have sufficient time for reflection and analysis. . . . Only if top management explicitly frees up employee time for this purpose does learning occur with any regularity" (p. 130). With all this focus on thinking, reflection, and analysis, it makes us wonder if all 17 of our dimensions could be found if we scrutinized that report.

Processes for Collecting, Monitoring, and Analyzing Errors

Organizations that are conscious entities operate as living organisms needing to be fed (Wheatley, 1994). Information is their food, "informatics" is the grocery store, and CT is the digestive system for the organization, allowing the information to be transformed into usable knowledge. To extend our analogy, we need to look at the "grocery carts" or devices used to collect the information we want transformed.

Some devices used by the experts to collect data include "root cause analysis," "near miss analysis," and "adverse events analysis" (IOM, 2004a). Once data are collected, CT is used to determine what to monitor and how to analyze the errors leading to safety gaps.

"Root cause analysis" is an earlier version of error identification strategies. This analysis searched for underlying causes and/or system failures that contributed to errors. The major problem with root cause analysis is that it is done after the fact and is considered to be too subjective. There is little evidence of its value in actually reducing errors (AHRQ, 1999). Yet the analysis continues to be used for tracking errors.

"Near miss analysis" examines data about situations that were caught before they happened—the errors. The IOM identified three goals for near miss analysis: 1) modeling (gaining qualitative insight into these types of errors), 2) trending (gaining quantitative insight into the patterns of errors), and 3) mindfulness (maintaining a high level of alertness to dangers). Unfortunately "near miss analysis" data are not routinely collected throughout the U.S. Only two states, Pennsylvania and Kansas, require near miss reporting (IOM, 2004a).

The purposes of "adverse event analysis" are to define events that need investigating, design ways to detect the events, and determine what data should be collected. Adverse event analyses help identify events labeled as "iatrogenic injuries." The major problem associated with adverse event analysis is that most events are not reported. The IOM (2004a) recommended three areas for improvement: 1) automated surveillance systems to capture the data, 2) more research to determine the effectiveness of the monitoring, and 3) integration of the data collection systems with patient care standards.

We have designed an adverse event analysis guideline to emphasize the thinking that is useful in analyzing errors. See Box 10.3 for the guidelines needed to complete TACTICS 10.5.

TACTICS 10.5 Thinking Through an Adverse Event

Clinicians and Educators

1. Ask nurses or students to record the details of a patient safety incident, paying particular attention to what they were thinking. To maintain anonymity, if that is desired, have those reports typed without names. Even better, have the event voice recorded so verbal nuances can be heard.
2. Give the incident to other nurses to analyze in terms of the CT dimensions.
3. Use the guidelines in Box 10.3 to help with that analysis. If several nurses analyze the same event, the total scores can be compared.
4. Discuss the how and why of each score.

Discussion

How did you and/or your colleagues do? Were you consistent in your scoring? In the event recorded, what CT dimensions were strong and could be enhanced? Consider how you could modify this guideline to fit your practice setting or course content. How can you use this to help emphasize the CT needed to improve safe care?

Safety Goals

Developing safety goals was recommended by the IOM (2004a) as a major step in improving safety. JCAHO has moved quickly in that area by establishing Patient Safety Goals for 10 healthcare settings, including hospitals ("National Patient Safety Goals for 2005 and 2004," n.d.).

Goals for Critical Access Hospitals for 2005, for example, as established by JCAHO are:

Box 10.3

Guidelines for Analyzing CT in an Event

Directions: Circle the number that best represents your conclusion.
2 = Yes, 1= Maybe, 0 = No

1. Was the nurse confident in his/her reasoning?   2 1 0
2. Was the whole situation (relationships, background, environment) taken into consideration?   2 1 0
3. Was there adequate consideration of alternatives, even those that were nontraditional or creative?   2 1 0
4. Was the nurse flexible enough?   2 1 0
5. Was the nurse engaged enough to really want to understand fully?   2 1 0
6. Were decisions based on usual practice and/or bias or was the truth sought even if it went contrary to usual practice?   2 1 0
7. Were there any intuitive signs of this happening?
8. Were all views considered? (The field was not narrowed too quickly.)   2 1 0
9. Did the nurse keep trying to solve the problem?   2 1 0
   (Didn't give up too quickly.)
10. Was there evidence of anyone standing back and reflecting on what was happening?   2 1 0
11. Was there evidence of the nurse breaking the situation down to better understand what was happening?   2 1 0
12. Were applicable standards upheld?   2 1 0
13. Were similarities or differences among parts of the issue distinguished carefully?   2 1 0
14. Was all possible information gathered?   2 1 0
15. Was there adequate evidence to support the conclusions drawn?   2 1 0
16. Was there evidence that this incident could have been predicted?   2 1 0
17. Was knowledge applied well in this situation?   2 1 0

                                                     Total Score:

Interpret Score

  0–15: Deficient CT probably contributed to event.

16–25: Insufficient CT possibly contributed to event.

26–30: CT may be insufficient but consider additional contributing factors.

31–34: CT was good; consider other contributing factors.

1. Improve the accuracy of patient identification.
2. Improve the effectiveness of communication among caregivers.
3. Improve the safety of using medications.
4. Improve the safety of using infusion pumps.
5. Reduce the risk of healthcare-associated infections.
6. Accurately and completely reconcile medications across the continuum of care.
7. Reduce the risk of patient harm resulting from falls ("2005 Critical Access Hospitals' National Patient Safety Goals," n.d.).

These and JCAHO's patient safety goals for other healthcare settings require "informatics" to collect (*information seeking*), monitor and interpret the aggregate data (*analysis* and *logical reasoning*), think about underlying system problems (*reflection* and *inquisitiveness*), and develop strategies to achieve safety goals (*flexibility, creativity, transforming knowledge, intuition, contextual perspective, perseverance,* and so forth). You get the picture.

IOM CRITERION #5

#5 Both act as an effective member of the interdisciplinary team and improve the quality of one's own performance through self assessment and personal change (IOM, 2003, p. 59).

This last criterion addresses CT directly, as it refers to self-assessment or *reflection.* As you will recall from Chapter 2, *reflection* is one of the 10 CT habits of the mind and was defined as "contemplation upon a subject, especially one's assumptions, and thinking for the purposes of deeper understanding and self evaluation" (Scheffer & Rubenfeld, 2000, p. 358).

The standard version of self-assessment (*reflection*) is typically done independently. *Reflection* encourages us to look back at our actions, behaviors, biases, and faulty reasoning. *Reflection* helps us find things we missed, consider things we want to work on differently, see patterns we did not recognize initially, wonder about solutions we did not consider at the time, and yes, even celebrate when our thinking was brilliant! ☺

But self-assessment is enhanced when it is validated by thinking and input from other perspectives. Brookfield (1995) identified four lenses or sources of feedback for *reflection:* autobiography, theory, students, and colleagues. Each lens is considered to have equal value during reflection. Each lens provides the educator or clinician with another point of view from which he or she can make comparisons and see patterns that confirm or discount what one or more of the other lenses reflects.

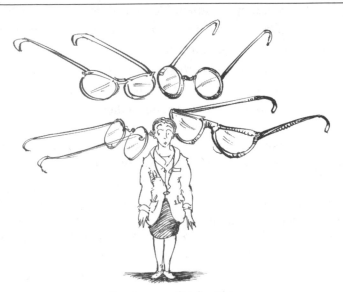

Four Lenses of Reflection

Self-assessment for Educators and Clinicians

Brookfield's four lenses of reflection can easily be used by educators or clinicians. Scenario 10.5 describes a shortened version of the clinician's use of the four lenses.

Scenario 10.5
Using Four Lenses for Reflection

Carol has been the nurse manager on an inpatient 24-bed psychiatric unit for the last three months. She has been trying to implement changes in interdisciplinary team work and wonders why the staff show little interest or do not follow through on plans after each staff meeting. She decides to do some reflection to better understand what is happening. Over the course of the next couple weeks, she uses all four lenses.

Autobiographical Lens: Carol considered herself a facilitative leader and promoter of collaboration. She took a continuing education course in leadership last year and went back to her notes to check off all the things the course recommended. She was doing them. From her perspective she was doing all the right things.

Patient/Staff Lens: Carol asked some staff what they thought about her leadership. They told her she was doing a great job. It *appeared the staff thought she was doing well but she wondered if they were just being nice. She didn't ask patients.*

Theoretical Lens: *Carol decided she would get on the Internet and got more undated information on management and leadership. She found others who are having similar problems with getting changes made. Carol found extensive information about management and about Interdisciplinary Teams. She read the management material, tried to schedule meetings more conveniently, and gave the staff copies of all she downloaded about Interdisciplinary Teams.*

The results were the same. The staff was not following through.

Colleagues Lens: *Carol remembered she had one more lens to use. She asked a colleague to sit in on the next couple of meetings and give her feedback. After the third meeting the colleague's feedback included, "Have you ever noticed how often you interrupt your staff with your own ideas?" The colleague also suggested how Carol might assign staff to search out reasons why Interdisciplinary Team Work such as this would encourage their more active participation. Her colleague reminded her about the "Discovery Learning" workshop they attended.*

Self-*reflection*'s *multiple lenses* allow clinicians and educators to examine and think about their practice and teach more effectively and accurately. We must, however, consciously and actively create opportunities to combine our thinking with the thinking of colleagues, patients, students, and the best available evidence to achieve the level of self-assessment that will more accurately lead to quality improvement. Again, we believe the IOM would endorse this kind of *reflection* for clinicians as well as educators.

SUMMARY OF THE FIVE IOM CRITERIA FOR QUALITY IMPROVEMENT

Our journey of thinking through the five IOM criteria for quality improvement has only begun. (And you thought this was the end!) To achieve quality through safe, effective, and efficient care we need to continually reflect on these criteria and use all dimensions of our CT to make them a reality in practice. Educators must incorporate these criteria into curricula if future practitioners are to be able to effectively apply quality improvement strategies.

We have one last TACTICS to illustrate how CT, the five IOM criteria for achieving quality improvement, and the five IOM competencies all come together.

TACTICS 10.6 Quality Care through CT

Read the questions below and answer them as you read and reflect on Scenario 10.6.

1. Which of the 17 thinking dimensions were demonstrated in the scenario?
2. How did Jeff achieve the five IOM criteria for quality improvement?
3. Which of the five IOM competencies (patient-centered care, interdisciplinary care, evidence-based practice, informatics, and quality improvement, see Box 10.2) were demonstrated in the scenario? And how could you have improved on them?

Scenario 10.6
Quality Care Through Individual and Team Thinking

Jeff is a rural Parish nurse. His clinic, 200 miles from the nearest hospital, includes a team of nurses, social workers, a nurse practitioner, and physical therapists. Contact with the hospital is by phone, e-mail, and fax. Jeff was scheduled to visit Mr. Youngblood, a 30-year-old single farmer, on his first day home from the hospital, where he had a bowel resection for diverticulitis and has a temporary colostomy.

Faxed orders for an initial home visit were for colostomy care. It had been some time since he had done colostomy care so he got on the Internet to check for EBP guidelines and called the Wound Ostomy & Continence Nurses Society for their help. Based on the information he found and feedback from the team, he questioned the frequency of the ordered bowel irrigations. He contacted the doctor, explained his concerns, and the order was changed.

The social worker knew Mr. Youngblood and provided information about his healthcare beliefs and how much he values his privacy. The team will meet again after Jeff's first visit to modify and adjust care planning.

Mr. Youngblood lived about 50 miles from the clinic. He had no phone, but Jeff left a message at the hospital before discharge to tell him the visit would be in the afternoon of his day of discharge.

Based on past experience with patients in rural areas, Jeff stocked his truck with a variety of items, just in case there were some unexpected circumstances. He knew that not all homes had all the amenities needed for standard healthcare procedures. He made sure his cell phone was fully charged even though he was only able to use it when he was on the tops of the mountain ridges.

When Jeff arrived, he found Mr. Youngblood sitting on his porch. He was sleeping in his rocking chair and needed physical contact to be aroused. With permission, Jeff began his assessment with vital signs. Although he was still weak from surgery, the assessment indicated all systems were WNL, with the exception of elimination and possibly his hearing. Assessment of the home environment revealed no indoor plumbing and water was brought to the house daily from a nearby stream. The home itself was neat and clean and he had adequate food supplies. Mr. Youngblood still drives. His nearest neighbor is two miles away.

Mr. Youngblood convinced his physician to discharge him early as he believed he would heal more quickly at home with the fresh air and peace and quiet that did not exist in the hospital. Besides, he did not believe it was good to have young female nurses doing what needed to be done. Mr. Youngblood was also adamant that he can't be bothered by doing "all this colostomy stuff more than once a day" because he needed to be in the fields all day long. Jeff did not remind him that work in the fields was probably going to have to wait until his strength returned.

Encouraging Mr. Youngblood to help with the problem solving, they worked out a plan for colostomy care that respected Mr. Youngblood's dignity, personal preferences, and need for quality colostomy care. The plan included Jeff filling empty gallon milk cartons with spring water and bringing them to the house to use for irrigation. Due to inadequate lighting in the house, they worked out a plan to do the irrigations and dressing changes by the window that received the best morning light and used an old bucket from the barn for the irrigation waste.

Disposing of the waste in the bucket was a concern. Mr. Youngblood told him not to worry. Jeff had a feeling Mr. Youngblood, who was very independent all his life, would try to solve this on his own. Jeff returned to the barn and found an old wagon that still worked. Until his strength returned, Mr. Youngblood agreed to use the bucket in the house, take it outside to the wagon at the end of the porch and pull it to the outhouse to be dumped. Suspecting that Mr. Youngblood might still try to carry the bucket on his own, Jeff asked him to promise to use the wagon for at least the first few weeks. He reluctantly agreed. An extra couple of gallon water jugs were left by the outhouse for rinsing the bucket.

After returning to the office, Jeff realized that he had misread Mr. Youngblood's antibiotic prescription. He had read "iii" on the Rx as "ii" because of the fuzziness of the fax. He visited the next day to correct his error and notified the physician. Jeff told the team to pay close attention to faxed information in all future orders.

Mr. Youngblood's strength gradually returned, he did use the wagon for a week until he was stronger and able to carry the bucket, he continued to do safe colostomy care with no complications, and take the correct dosage of his antibiotic. His second surgery to reconnect his bowel was successful. Jeff continued to visit to monitor progress, working with the healthcare team and following Mr. Youngblood's preferences. Further assessment revealed that Mr. Youngblood was losing his hearing, but he refused suggestions for a hearing test. The team respected his wishes in spite of the increased risk to his safety while living alone.

Discussion

Thinking used:

Transforming knowledge was demonstrated when Jeff had to adjust what he knew were normal procedures for colostomy care in a hospital to the rural environment with fewer resources.

Confidence was demonstrated in challenging the physician's order for frequency of bowel irrigations.

Contextual perspective was demonstrated when Jeff assessed the home environment as well as Mr. Youngblood's healthcare beliefs and incorporated the input from the social worker.

Creativity was demonstrated when Jeff and Mr.Youngblood came up with several plans to use the available resources to achieve safe care.

Predicting was demonstrated when Jeff thought about the extra supplies he might need in a rural setting.

Intuition was demonstrated when Jeff suspected Mr. Youngblood would try to be too independent before his strength returned.

Five IOM Criteria for Achieving Quality Improvement:

#1 Jeff considered structure by taking into consideration Mr. Youngblood's preferences and his environment. He paid attention to process in his interactions with Mr. Youngblood and the other healthcare providers. He monitored outcomes in the form of Mr. Youngblood's tolerance for the medications, ability to stay infection–free, and ability to maintain a quality of life he preferred.

#2 Jeff assessed current practice and searched for better practice when he used the Internet and conferred with his colleagues for the best approaches.

#3 Jeff very creatively designed and monitored his interventions for effectiveness.

#4 Jeff identified his error and the defect in the fax system. He took steps to avoid this "adverse event" in the future.

#5 Jeff's scenario does not highlight reflection but we will assume he did so when he realized the medication error.

IOM Competencies addressed:

Patient-centered care was demonstrated when Jeff worked to meet Mr. Youngblood's desire to be home during his recovery and Jeff did not push Mr. Youngblood to follow up on his hearing loss after he preferred not to.

Interdisciplinary team work was demonstrated when Jeff consulted with the nursing team, the physician, and the social worker and together created a plan.

Evidence-based practice was demonstrated when Jeff searched the Internet for current guidelines for colostomy care.

Informatics utilization was demonstrated when Jeff used the Internet and the fax machine for information.

Applying quality improvement was demonstrated when Jeff provided safe, effective, and efficient care in Mr. Youngblood's home environment. He also applied quality improvement by recognizing a medication error, fixing the error, and addressing the system problem that created it.

PAUSE AND PONDER:
GUARDIANS OF QUALITY IMPROVEMENT

Well, here we are at the end of another important chapter. The current situation in healthcare with the number of deaths solely resulting from errors is not tolerable. Applying quality improvement thinking is mandatory. What will the future of quality improvement hold? How are you and other providers going to take up the challenge and become the guardians of quality improvement? *You* are the providers who will take care of us and our families (and your families) and educate future providers, so we have a vested interest in cultivating all of the CT necessary. We believe you are up to the challenge.

Reflection Cues

- "Quality is the degree to which health services for individuals and populations increase the likelihood of desired health outcomes and are consistent with current professional knowledge" (IOM, 1990, p. 4).
- Gaps in quality have led to as many as 98,000 deaths a year as a result of errors in healthcare.

- Quality assurance and CQI procedures are evolving to quality improvement procedures by re-focusing toward prevention of errors and identifying system problems as opposed to blaming individuals.
- Structure, process, and outcomes remain valuable concepts in healthcare but are more valuable when all three are looked at as a whole.
- Once we accept that errors will occur, we can constructively look for errors and hazards and realistically seek to improve safety for patients.
- "Near misses" and "adverse events" are frequently attributed to the poor design, communication patterns, and organization of the healthcare delivery system, not individuals.
- "Root cause analysis," "Near miss analysis," and "adverse event analysis" are three strategies for collecting the data necessary to improve systems to decrease errors.
- Changing the organizational culture to a "culture of safety" requires thinking from individuals, administration, and the interdisciplinary team to change values, attitudes, and beliefs about errors.
- Thinking remains the key to applying quality improvement in healthcare to achieve safe, effective, and efficient care.
- Matching the data with conclusions, matching the right provider to patient needs, and matching appropriate tests and procedures to patient conditions are essential aspects of effective care.
- Old beliefs and attitudes about perfection and avoiding errors severely limit our ability to collect accurate data for research and decisions on system changes.
- Improvements in quality require CT in both practice and education, focusing on the five IOM competencies, the five IOM criteria for quality, and all 17 dimensions of CT.

References

2005 Critical Access Hospitals' National Patient Safety Goals. (n.d.). Retrieved August 3, 2004, from http://www.jcaho.org/accredited+organizations/patient+safety/05+npsg/05_npsg_cah.htm.

Agency for Healthcare Research and Quality. (1999). *Making healthcare safer: A critical analysis of patient safety practices.* Rockville, MD: AHRQ.

Affonso, D. D. & Doran, D. (2002). Cultivating discoveries in patient safety research: A framework. *International Nursing Perspectives, 2*(1), 33–47.

Alemi, F. (1999). Continuous quality improvement: Cult or science counterpoint? *Nursing Leadership Forum, 4*(1), 5–8.

Benner, P. (2001). Creating a culture of safety and improvement: A key to reducing medical error. *American Journal of Critical Care, 10*(4), 281–284.

Brookfield, S. D. (1995). *Becoming a critically reflective teacher.* San Francisco: Jossey-Bass.

Donabedian, A. (2003). *An introduction to "quality assurance."* New York: Oxford University Press.

Facts about Patient Safety. (n.d.). Retrieved August 5, 2004, from (http://www.jcaho.org/accredited+organizations/patient+safety/facts+about+patient+safety.html).

Famous quotes, Einstein quotes. (n.d.). Retrieved August 1, 2004, from http://home.att.net/~quotations/einstein.html.

Gloe, D. (1998). Quality management: A staff development tradition. In K. J. Kelly-Thomas (Ed.) *Clinical and nursing staff development: Current competence, future focus.* (2nd ed.) (pp. 301–336.) Philadelphia: Lippincott.

Henneman, E. A. & Gawlinski, A. (2004). A "Near-Miss" Model for describing the nurse's role in the recovery of medical errors. *Journal of Professional Nursing, 20*(3), 1106–201.

Institute of Medicine. (1990). *Medicare: A strategy for quality assurance: Executive summary IOM committee to design a strategy for quality review and assurance in Medicare.* Washington, DC: The National Academies Press.

Institute of Medicine. (2000). *To err is human: Building a safer health system.* Washington, DC: The National Academies Press.

Institute of Medicine. (2001). *Crossing the quality chasm: A new health system for the 21st century.* Washington, DC: The National Academies Press.

Institute of Medicine. (2003). *Health professions education: A bridge to quality.* Washington, DC: The National Academies Press.

Institute of Medicine. (2004a). *Patient safety: Achieving a new standard for care.* Washington, DC: The National Academies Press.

Institute of Medicine. (2004b). *Keeping patients safe: Transforming the work environment of nurses.* Washington, DC: The National Academies Press.

Leape, L. L. (1994). Error in medicine. *Journal of the American Medical Association, 272,* 1851–1857.

National Patient Safety Goals for 2005 and 2004. (n.d.). Retrieved August 3, 2004, from http://jcaho.org/accredited+organizations/patient+safety/npsg.htm.

Plsek, P. (2003, January). *Complexity and the adoptions of innovation in healthcare.* Paper presented at the conference *Accelerating Quality Improvement in Healthcare Strategies to Speed the Diffusion of Evidence-based Innovations,* by National Institute for Healthcare Management Foundation and National Committee for Quality Healthcare, Washington, DC.

Pronovost, P. J. (2004, March). *Healthcare safety and quality revolution.* Presentation, the American Association of Colleges of Nursing Spring Annual Meeting, Fairmont Hotel, Washington, DC.

Scheffer, B. K. & Rubenfeld, M. G. (2000). A consensus statement on critical thinking in nursing. *Journal of Nursing Education, 39*(8), 352–359.

Sentinel Event ALERT. (July 21, 2004). Retrieved August 3, 2004, from http://www.jcaho.org/about+us/news+letters/sentinel+event+alert/print/sea_30.htm.

Shortell, S. M., Bennett, C. L., & Byck, G. R. (1998). Assessing the impact of continuous quality improvement on clinical practice: What it will take to accelerate progress. *The Milbank Quarterly, 76*(4), 5103–624.

This Month at the Joint Commission. (2004, July). Retrieved August 3, 2004, from http://www.jcaho.org/about+us/news+letters/this+month/print/july+2004.htm.

Westrum, R. & Gleason, S. C. (2003). A culture of patient safety. *AHRQ User Liaison Program.* Retrieved October 16, 2003, from http://www.arq.gov/news/ulp/ptsafety/ptsafety2.htm.

Wheatley, M. J. (1994). *Leadership and the new science: Learning about organization from an orderly universe.* San Francisco: Berrett-Koehler Publishers.

CHAPTER 11

Thinking Realities of Yesterday, Today, and Tomorrow

Here we are at the other bookend chapter for our discussions of thinking with the five competencies—patient-centered care, working in interdisciplinary teams, using evidence-based practice, using informatics, and achieving quality improvement. We introduced these IOM (2003) competencies in Chapter 5 as we put the *how*, *where*, and *when* of CT together and suggested some active teaching/learning approaches for educators and strategies for reflection in practice for clinicians. Now, we step back to look at what all this means to our day-to-day existence as healthcare providers and educators. This existence is certainly not what it used to be ten, or even five years ago. We are working in a different world today. As to any significance of this being "Chapter Eleven," we hope our thinking won't be so taxed that we go bankrupt!! (It's OK to groan at that.) An overwhelming theme throughout the last six chapters has been change. In Box 11.1 we've summarized the change messages in those chapters to refresh your memory.

The inevitability of change in healthcare right now is a timely topic these days. Statements like these abound: "The U.S. healthcare system requires radical, not incremental, change" (Waldman, Smith, & Hood, 2003, p. 5). "It's the end of an era. The type of nursing learned by the average, 47-year-old nurse is ending" (Porter-O'Grady, 2003, p. 4). We will discuss the thinking needed to deal with these changes shortly, but first let's reflect on why change is so necessary in healthcare right now and the implications of that constant, complex change to our daily existence.

WHY IS CHANGE SO NECESSARY?

The answers to why change is necessary right now are all around us. Read any newspaper and you'll see articles on problems with healthcare systems and the health of people around us—our ill-prepared plans to deal with the increased numbers of elderly patients with multiple health conditions, the huge increase in Type 2 diabetes in young people, the high rate of obesity, our ability to keep people alive without quality of life, potential deadly outbreaks of new and mutated microorganisms, the imbalance between infinite needs and

Box 11.1

Evolving Themes of Change in Chapters 6–10

From . . .	Provider-centered care	to . . .	Patient-centered care
From . . .	Giving patients information	to . . .	Coaching patients to find information
From . . .	Present patient needs/tasks	to . . .	Future patient needs/tasks
From . . .	Multidisciplinary work	to . . .	Interdisciplinary teamwork
From . . .	Individual perspective	to . . .	Contextual perspective
From . . .	Individual CT	to . . .	Team/System CT
From . . .	Dichotomous thinking	to . . .	Relativistic thinking
From . . .	Tradition-based practice	to . . .	Evidence-based practice
From . . .	Change based on anecdotes	to . . .	Change based on strong evidence
From . . .	Paper and pens	to . . .	Informatics
From . . .	Information	to . . .	Knowledge
From . . .	Quality assurance	to . . .	Quality improvement
From . . .	Culture of blame for errors	to . . .	Culture of safety
From . . .	Status quo	to . . .	Innovation
From . . .	Hierarchical power	to . . .	Empowerment of all professionals

finite resources, the shortage of nurses and nurse educators, the high rates of medical errors, the rapid growth of new medications and treatment possibilities, antibiotic resistance, and . . . shall we keep going?

By the way, as an aside for you educators, we'll share a tactic we use in many of our courses—assignments to increase students' awareness of local to global health issues that are in the news. We have students find articles from the popular media and discuss their implications for nurses. It is always an eye-opening project because many students perceive nurses as dealing with one patient at a time. We are trying to get them better socialized to the many issues that will force them to be changeable and adaptable in their careers.

The examples we listed above are areas needing change specifically in healthcare delivery, but remember, according to the IOM those changes need to start in the health education arena. We are not only talking about the complex changes in healthcare, we are also talking about complex educational change. Changes in educational systems may be even harder to realize because of the traditions. As Senge, Scharmer, Jaworski, and Flowers (2004) pointed out, our present educational system is based on industrial-age assembly-line principles that will not prepare people to deal with tomorrow's realities. We health educators have a double whammy to deal with; we cannot escape change either in the classroom or in the clinical settings.

WHAT KINDS OF CHANGE ARE WE TALKING ABOUT?

There have been zillions of books, articles, monographs, and so forth written on the change process and strategies to implement and deal with change. Those that are relevant to healthcare delivery and education start with descriptions of change that depict the confounding complexity of systems such as ours. Paul Plsek presented a thoughtful, practical perspective for a conference convened in Washington, DC by the National Institute for Health Care Management Foundation and the National Committee for Quality Health Care (2003). Plsek focused on change in healthcare as a complex issue, making a distinction between complex, complicated, and simple issues. Change in healthcare is complex because the healthcare system is a complex adaptive system. "A complex adaptive system is a collection of individual agents who have the freedom to act in ways that are not always totally predictable, and whose actions are interconnected such that one agent's actions change the context for other agents" (Plsek, 2003, Second Section, "Health Care as a Complex").

Models for complex adaptive systems are organic systems such as the human body—where a change in one part will affect a change in another and where it must always be viewed as a whole, not a collection of parts. In these systems, while there are feedback mechanisms to maintain the status quo, there is always something changing; there are contradictions and lots of unknowns. Think of what happens with a sore knee. To ease the knee, a person changes his gait and gets hip or foot pain, takes medications such as NSAIDS for the pain, and gets side effects of edema that aggravate hypertension. A simple sore knee now presents a potential cardiac problem. We would do well to keep that image in mind when we start to consider complex system changes.

Other authors have made distinctions between types of complexity—detailed and/or dynamic (Senge, 1990). The latter, dynamic complexity, is what we see in healthcare—the very nature of the complexity is focused on change. Senge et al. (2004) recently discussed this as transformational change, which is highly focused on the people involved in the change, not just on what and how the change is made. It must focus on who we are. "The changes in which we will be called upon to participate in the future will be both deeply personal and inherently systemic" (p. 2). People transform systems; systems don't transform themselves.

Educational systems and change are equally complex, according to Fullan (1993). "Complexity, dynamism, and unpredictability . . . are not merely things that get in the way. They are normal" (p. 20). Many processes are unknowable in advance and there is nothing linear about the complexities of educational systems and their change. Making educational change more paradoxical is that, while change is a continuous theme, the educational system is essentially conservative. Change in these circumstances cannot occur through isolated reforms; the whole educational system needs to become a "learning organization—expert at dealing with change as a normal part of its work . . ." (Fullan, 1993, p. 4).

Linear thinking about change as going from data to conclusions, mandates to coercion, chaos to order, and so forth is facile, revealing unrealistic thinking processes for today's changes in these complex systems. Fullan (1993) advocated better thinking as a solution. "The solution lies in better ways of thinking about, and dealing with, inherently unpredictable processes" (p. 19). Among his eight basic lessons for this new paradigm of change are three of our favorites: "You can't mandate what matters. . . . Connection with the wider environment is critical for success . . . [and] every person is a change agent" (pp. 21–22). These lessons emphasize the involvement of everyone in this thinking journey. In a little while we'll discuss the changes in thinking that need to accompany the changes in healthcare delivery and education. First, however, we must consider the reactions of people involved in change.

IMPLICATIONS OF LIVING WITH CONSTANT, COMPLEX CHANGE

What about the implications of living with constant, let alone complex, change? With change comes the certainty of uncertainty, messiness, excitement, challenges, learning, refining self, redefining positions, more interactions among people, and calls for creativity. With change comes the possibility (probability?) of coercion, increased work, fatigue, anger, anxiety, judgments, feelings of inadequacy, and a desire to "run away." It's all pretty scary stuff, right? How can we survive with our wits intact in this kind of changing day-to-day reality? For starters we have to reflect on how we view change and the kinds of experiences we've had with change in the past. Then we have to look at how that view fits with the thinking needed today.

So, just what have been your experiences with change? Many (most?) clinicians and educators have negative experiences. Changes have been handed down from upper-level administration and management. Before we can settle into one change, another comes along to take its place. Sometimes that happens even before we've settled into the first change! People far removed from the day-to-day implementation of the change developed the plan without our input. Before we feel comfortable with the change we are being evaluated on how well we are doing with it. The focus is on the endpoint of the change rather than the process of change. Many changes are instigated to save money. Money-saving changes often have a short- rather than long-term goal. Many changes seem irrelevant or were tried and found ineffective in other situations. Every time we hear from our manager that something is about to change, we feel anxiety!

This hierarchical system, with rapidly increasing frequency of episodic change, has been the norm for nurses for a long time. We need to acknowledge that, reflect on it, think about the feelings it brings up, and then think about how we can deal with it successfully in the future.

THINKING FOR EFFECTIVE CHANGE

The old ways of thinking about change won't work any longer. "As long as our thinking is governed by habit—notably by industrial, 'machine age' concepts such as control, predictability, standardization, and 'faster is better'—we will continue to re-create institutions as they have been, despite their increasing disharmony with the larger world" (Senge et al., 2004, p. 5).

Figure 11.1   Realities of Thinking

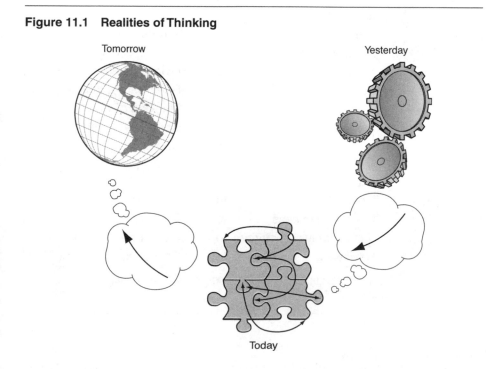

Tomorrow

Yesterday

Today

As we consider the critical thinking dimensions that are our model in this book, once again we can look at all 17 and see how integral they are to the change process. We have addressed all of them in the last five chapters as we've discussed changes inherent in thinking about the five competencies. However, here we'd like to examine six dimensions that are especially important in dealing with the complex, dynamic change that is needed and inevitable. We will focus on *contextual perspective, creativity, intuition, inquisitiveness, reflection,* and *transforming knowledge.* It's not that the others aren't used or important, it's just that these six are particularly useful in helping us initiate and deal with change.

We aren't really going to separate these six very much either because they are so interrelated. What we've done instead is list 15 patterns of change in thinking and learning that, from our review of literature and collective experience, require an amalgamation of these several dimensions. See Box 11.2.

Box 11.2

Emergent, Necessary Patterns of Change in Thinking and Learning

1. From . . .	Passivity	to . . .	Engagement/Presence
2. From . . .	Answers	to . . .	Questions
3. From . . .	Separate thinking and doing	to . . .	Thinking and doing together
4. From . . .	Destination	to . . .	Journey
5. From . . .	Reactive learning	to . . .	Proactive learning
6. From . . .	Mechanistic models	to . . .	Living system models
7. From . . .	Dichotomous thinking	to . . .	Relativistic thinking
8. From . . .	Thinking of pieces	to . . .	Thinking of wholes
9. From . . .	Alone/Separated	to . . .	Connected/Systems
10. From . . .	Reduction	to . . .	Complexity
11. From . . .	Matching existing patterns	to . . .	New patterns
12. From . . .	Linear	to . . .	Maps/Knots/Shapes
13. From . . .	Constant success	to . . .	Failure possibilities
14. From . . .	Valuing only objectivity	to . . .	Being open to intuition
15. From . . .	Reviewing	to . . .	Reflecting

(References: Senge, 1998, 2004; Senge et al., 2004; Plsek & Greenhalgh, 2001; Plsek, 2003; Porter-O'Grady, 2003; Fullan, 1993)

EMERGENT, NECESSARY PATTERNS
OF CHANGE IN THINKING AND LEARNING

Today's reality just doesn't fit with yesterday's thinking patterns. We are not dealing with a machine; we are dealing with a complex system of human beings that is intertwined with many other systems, all in a state of constant flux. As Senge et al. (2004) and Plsek (2003) noted, much of our thinking about organizations has come from the industrial age and a mechanistic mentality that favors assembly lines. Modern systems like healthcare don't work that way; they are adaptive, with complex feedback mechanisms. If we want to successfully change healthcare we have to approach it more like a living organism system than a machine. (Remember our knee example earlier.) Of course, as soon as we move to the living system metaphor, we can see that, in contrast to machine systems, there is very little predictability and a whole lot of potential chaos. As clinicians and educators, not only do we need to initiate change ourselves, we must survive changes instigated by others. For that, we've developed these 15 patterns of change in thinking and learning in Box 11.2. We added learning because today's systems are learning environments, not just places to do things.

From Passivity to Engagement/Presence

We have to see that this inevitable change will affect us, but we also have to see that we will affect that change as well. It is not a one-way, but a two-way street. No longer can we sit back and let someone tell us what to do. We have a long tradition of learning and thinking in this passive mode. Educators keep presenting lectures; students keep reading, underlining, memorizing, and spitting back. Clinicians, toward the end of this chapter we tell the story of a nurse who epitomized engagement in introducing and working through a change. If you don't already have an active approach to your job, think about what it would take to make you more engaged in thinking about changes that are necessary and how you might instigate those changes. Look back to Chapter 5 at the suggestions for reflection in action to increase your engagement. Educators, look back, also, to Chapter 5 and think about your teaching styles (Box 5.6 on page 91). Are you promoting passive or active learning? If you are continuing this passive tradition, you are not helping students prepare for the reality they will face. You have to risk getting some bad evaluations while trying different active strategies because students are pretty stuck in their passive learning modes. Most have come through passive educational systems where they've been taught there is one "right" answer.

From Answers to Questions

Because change is constant with many issues, unknown until they evolve, there are fewer answers, especially simple ones and, for sure, there is not just one right answer. Senge said, "Genuine inquiry starts when people ask questions to which they do not have an answer" (1998, np, section 4). Focusing on questions keeps the door to change open. Remember our discussion of Problem-Based Learning in Chapter 5? The core of that approach is starting with a problem or a question to guide learning (Rideout, 2001). Creative people ask questions: How can I represent the best aesthetic placement of these flowers? Why is this happening? What will this patient need to adapt at home? Later in this chapter we tell one nurse's story of innovative practice that started with a question: Why are we seeing deep sternal infections post-operatively?

We tend to focus more on answers because it's neater. Think of how much better most people feel after they've straightened up their homes, closets, workbenches, or desks. For a brief period, we have a sense of order in what is increasingly a disorderly world. Questioning takes us down a path of ambiguity because it allows for the possibility that the world isn't perfect. But, of course, the world isn't perfect, especially healthcare practice and education. We really do need to change things, so let's get rid of that desire for perfection, step out into the uncertainty, and question everything, especially those things for which we don't already have answers.

From Separate Thinking and Doing to Thinking and Doing Together

A class activity that we have used for many years at the start of our critical thinking course is to have students draw their "thinking caps." You may want to try this tactic; it's a great CT discussion initiator. After the initial, "*What* do you want?" questions, students get enough reassurance to draw their caps. The results are quite interesting. Some talk about putting on a "hat" and going some place quiet and peaceful to think. They tend to have neat hats with brims. Other students have pictures of things that could only be called "hats" by the most creative; they have all kinds of things going on at once and they discuss how everything is open and accessible. Secretly we think, "Ah, they'll be better able to adapt to thinking in nursing," but we never say that of course; we wait for them to see that as the semester progresses, and they broaden their thinking as they see their peers' hats and hear them described.

Now, why do you think we see the latter group of students as being more adaptable to nurse thinking? It's because their thinking is all tied up with their doing, their emotions, things in their lives. They don't picture their thinking in neat, safe, clean spaces; therefore thinking in the midst of the chaos of healthcare situations will not be a shock to them and they will likely have an easier time doing *reflection* in practice.

You might want to *reflect* on when and how you do your thinking. Do you tend to sit back and do it after the fact or while you're actively doing something?

From Destinations to Journeys

This is similar to moving from answers to questions because it's about uncertainty and ambiguity. We tend to think about our end points. Things will be better once I get the kitchen fixed; we'll have more money once the kids have finished school; I'll get some order back in my life once the semester ends. This kind of thinking actually sets us up for frustration because, of course, in today's complex world, almost nothing goes into a neat box upon which we can write "finished." Just ask people about projects they have that have never gotten finished; ask them how they feel about them. You'll find some who say, "This is just how life is; I always have things unfinished and I've learned to live with it." Others are bothered by the lack of closure and try endlessly to close boxes.

Healthcare service and education will never be "finished" with their changes because every change will affect something else that will have to change. New technology will come along and redefine even the simple things that we have firmly in place and we'll have to open boxes all too frequently. Accept that, start to look more at the journey than the destination, and you'll be less crazy in this world.

If you want a hard lesson in the journey versus destination thinking, write an article or a book and you'll realize how hard it is to let it go as a finished product. As soon as you send it off to the publisher, you read something that you wish you had addressed. That's, of course, why you should always cite authors in the past tense. There's a good chance they might not say today what they said last year!

From Reactive Learning to Proactive Learning

This, too, is related to the first patterns we discussed—to move from passivity to engagement and from answers to questions—but we feel it's worth describing in these alternate terms to make sure this whole idea comes through. Senge et al. (2004) described reactive learning as "governed by 'downloading' habitual ways of thinking, of continuing to see the world within the familiar categories we're comfortable with. . . . At best, we get better at what we have always done" (p. 6). They made a distinction between "reactive" and "deeper" learning, but we've chosen to call the other end of the pattern "proactive" learning, which we think becomes "deeper" because learners are much more involved in seeking knowledge and putting it into a better workable frame for themselves.

How much of what you read is because someone told you to read it or recommended it to you? How does that compare to what you read because you were curious enough to go digging something out yourself? How many of you, when you were students, read the recommended readings in addition to the required ones? Ahem, did we strike a nerve there?

When you meet someone new, how much do you ask about what they do and try to learn from them? We have a friend, Connie, and everywhere she goes she asks tons of questions of everyone she meets. If you happen to be tagging along, you might get antsy as she gets deeper and deeper into conversations, oblivious to time. She is very bright and knows a lot about a lot of things and has worked as a writer/reporter for many years. We're not sure if this is a chicken or egg thing—if she became a writer because she was so curious and wanted to share her knowledge, or if she became that way from being assigned to stories. It's probably a bit of both—just a good match. What she is, without a doubt, is a proactive learner—so much so that she made a guilt-free decision not to finish her doctoral dissertation because it became too narrow a focus for her and she didn't want to endorse that type of learning!

So where are you, compared to Connie? Most of us are more reactive. We go along with the reactive-learning model of mainstream education and many of us promote reactive learning in our students. It's tough to give up the power of teacher teaching to the power of the learner's learning, but we educators have to move more in that direction if we are to coach active, creative innovators in healthcare. Remember Fullan's (1993) lesson number one: you can't mandate what matters. Learners need to come to their learning proactively to be invested in what they are learning and achieve deeper understanding as a result.

From Mechanistic Models to Living Systems Models

We discussed this earlier when we described the types of change needed today. What about the thinking involved in this change of perspective? This is "running like clockwork." We have a "well-oiled machine here." Even though we use such metaphors, do we really believe that our healthcare and education systems fit that picture? Probably not. Senge (1998, 2004) repeatedly pointed out the need to consider living systems as our model of change in today's complex world. A most important lesson we have learned from his writings is to consider the impact of compensating feedback mechanisms in living systems and how that differs from the workings of machines. If you've ever dieted to lose weight (and who hasn't?) you can relate. Initially you lose weight and then you gain a bit and/or level off even when you think you're eating the same way. Your body is hanging on to your "survival" fat and has a starvation feedback signal. Some of us try to reset that thermostat periodically, some with more success than others, by changing our eating and activity patterns. Much of the resistance to change that we observe is the system trying to conserve itself or something within itself. If we don't recognize the process or what it is trying to conserve, we will continue to be frustrated with "resistance to change."

Senge (1998, 2004) used the example of a hot room with a thermostat. You enter and, without knowledge of the thermostat, you open the windows to cool things off. Soon it gets warmer again. If you want change, you have to get to the thermostat and reset it or turn off the furnace. Think about that image the next time you wonder why your group is hanging on to something and doesn't want to change; figure out where the furnace is or figure out how to reset the thermostat. Translate that to what the group is hanging on to and what will change their value of that.

From Dichotomous Thinking to Relativistic Thinking

OK, this is all about *contextual perspective*, right? Is there anyone still out there who sees things clearly in terms of right or wrong, blue or yellow, yes or no? We'd like to think that all of you would say, "Well, that depends." And that's the answer that goes "chi-ching" on the relativistic side. Of course, we know all clinicians and educators don't say that, and those who do acknowledge they only do it sometimes. Hey, have you taken a multiple-choice test lately? Better yet, have you given one? What do you do with the student who is arguing with this line—well, what about if this . . .?

One of the great education ironies in nursing is that we try and try to promote relativistic thinking in students so they'll look at the whole context of a clinical situation, but then we test them with dichotomous exams that have rigid right or wrong answers. Because we still have to prepare students for multiple choice licensure exams, even those of us who hate such exams feel pressure to allow some practice with them. We've gotten around our discomfort with this dichotomous approach by allowing students to challenge questions and answers. "If you can show in writing that your answer is as good as mine, you get credit for that question." It's not the best lesson in relativistic thinking, but it lets us sleep at night.

From Thinking of Pieces to Thinking of Wholes

It is very easy to focus on the tree in front of you and forget about the forest, but, because living systems are so interconnected, it is folly to be too narrow in your view. Think about how short patient stays in hospital are these days. Recently, in a class of RNs we asked about patient teaching and several students replied that they rarely do any patient teaching because they worked in ICUs—that this was something done more by the nurses "on the floors." Needless to say I raised my eyebrows a bit and asked questions like this: Don't your patients have family members sitting around? How often are your patients discharged home only a day or two after leaving the ICU? What constitutes patient teaching to you? Ultimately, the students realized they were working in a very task-oriented way and were not seeing the whole picture of these patients' lives and how this episode of illness fit within it. They realized that there were lots of "little" things that they could and should be teaching to patients and to family members.

How are we going to get past that task orientation that has been such a huge part of our history in nursing? Educators, how can we teach novices who are so focused on tasks to periodically look up and see the whole patient? One idea is to start teaching tasks with more focus on the absolute essential parts so that students can stop using up their RAM with unnecessary details, leaving more of their hard drives open for bigger pictures. We can also pepper our check-off routines with "What if . . ." questions to get them thinking of this task in a large, constantly changing context.

Clinicians, look around you at things like end-of-shift reports and count how many times a larger view of patients' worlds is mentioned. Start modeling that yourself. Put something in your report room to remind nurses of the larger view—a globe or a picture of a family picnic.

From Thinking Alone to Systems Thinking

This theme is especially emphasized in Chapter 7, on interdisciplinary teams. While we need to hone our individual thinking skills, we have to also focus on how we think as groups. Carole Estabrooks (2003) presented a view of nurses within communities of practice. On first reading we feared we would have trouble getting nurses to move to new thinking approaches, such as evidence-based practice (EBP). However, her remarks proved worthy of reflection beyond our first reactions. Here's what she found: "Increasingly, we are aware that nurses rely more on knowledge generated within their communities of practice than on knowledge generated by research. In particular, we have found that 'social interactions' and 'experience' are the two most important sources of knowledge for nurses . . . learning is social" (pp. 60–61). From that perspective, group thinking is perhaps already in place in nursing practice. Estabrooks acknowledged that this social learning phenomenon needs to be studied more, and we agree with her.

If we assume that Estabrooks is on to something, maybe we're halfway there in increasing our group or systems thinking. Maybe we're closer to systems thinking in nursing than professionals are in some other disciplines. Perhaps we should put our energies into the type of learning and thinking that is occurring in those social interactions. To continue with our EBP example, if a group of nurses is using traditions as a basis for practice, then we need to target that group and encourage some of them to explore EBP. All it takes is an instigation of social interactions around a new evidence report or a question about a practice that all nurses can relate to. This is the place for the clinician who models CT, talks aloud about thinking, and asks lots of questions.

From Reduction to Complexity

We probably have our logical positivist tradition to thank for our penchant for reductionist thinking. While analysis and reducing problems to discover and learn are definite assets to CT, we have to take care that we put things back together after we've done that reduction. This is an issue that comes up when trying to explain critical thinking. It is so complex that we have to break it down to make it understandable; hence the 17 dimensions. However, as you can probably see by now, each time we try to address each dimension separately it is never clean. These dimensions work best in harmony, as a whole where they augment each other.

Educators need to be especially aware of complex new patterns of change; years ago we used to be able to teach in a reductionist manner—break everything down so students can understand the pieces. However, students are left with skills that they can't put into use because nothing in the clinical world is reduced in that way. Educators must help students put the pieces back together to see the enormous complexity that is the setting for these reduced skills.

From Matching Existing Patterns to New Patterns

When we see something new, we tend to interpret and store it in the established patterns in our brains. It's easier to remember something when it's in the form of a familiar pattern (Hart, 1983). An old pattern might be used to process and store something you hear your manager say—"I want everyone to be involved in coming up with ideas for improvement." If the usual style of change on your unit is hierarchical, with edicts handed down from above, that old pattern for registering the manager's remark might be, "That means we should all be nice and go along with things." It is very hard to throw off old patterns and make new ones. It means standing back and looking at things with "different" eyes. It doesn't necessarily mean throwing away the old patterns; it might be easier sometimes just to change the shape of the existing ones.

Plsek (2003) gave a great example of creative thinking in new connections of patterns to help us teach patients better. We know that repetition helps learning; we know that elderly patients and those under stress often forget things we teach them; we know that, if we could tape record what we tell patients, they could go back and listen to it again; we know that most people have telephone answering machines. The new pattern then, is to put all of those existing patterns together and come up with a plan to record our teaching on patients' home answering machines while we teach them face-to-face. We just ask them if we can call their homes and record the teaching session. Then they can, when they get home, listen to it as often as needed.

These ideas are often called thinking outside the box; some people are better at it than others. In today's world of change we all must get outside our boxes and open ourselves to new patterns. To tease your brain a bit, look at Box 11.3; see if you can figure out these puzzles. The first one was brought home from school by one of our sons and we're not sure who created it. We both had trouble with it, even though it's very simple, because we have moved to thinking patterns where numbers are things we count, add, subtract, multiply with, and so forth. We don't look at numbers as words and that's the key to figuring out that pattern. Have you figured it out yet? The next line is 312211—Three ones, two twos, and one one. Start at the top now and say the words instead of seeing the numbers; one one—two ones—one two and one one, and so on.

The second example is from a wonderful book by Harvard's David Perkins (1994) on learning to think by looking at art. In a chapter called "Making Looking Broad and Adventurous" he presented that number puzzle. Once again, one

---

Box 11.3

Brain Teasers To Help Develop/Use New Brain Patterns

The First Example:

1

11

21

1211

111221

What is the next line?

The Second Example (Perkins, 1994):

$2 + 7 - 118 = 129$

Add one straight line to the mathematical statement above to make it true instead of false. There are at least three solutions.

has to get away from usual patterns and assumptions to see the possible solutions. The first solution is to put a vertical line through the equals sign. Did you just say, "duh"? The second solution is to put a line starting at the left end of the top part of the equals sign and extend it diagonally up to the right. This creates the sign meaning less than or equals and makes the statement true also. The third solution is different; with one line on the plus sign, you make it into a four and then the equation becomes $247 - 118 = 129$. As Perkins explained, we tend not to cut across categories in our minds. We tend to see things in habitual patterns.

From Linear to Maps/Knots/Shapes

There is nothing linear about the thinking necessary for initiating and dealing with change in complex adaptive systems. Looking for straight lines just sets us up for frustration. Linear thinking does not allow us to be contextual and see the whole. We don't even have neat circles and ovals with today's thinking; we have varying shapes such as knots, where things are so interconnected that it's hard to separate the pieces.

There are many resources in nursing today advocating mind or concept maps as learning mechanisms (e.g., Mueller, Johnston, & Bligh, 2002; Novak, 1998; Wheeler & Collins, 2003). We have been using them for clinical courses in place of columnar care plans, critical thinking classes to show nonlinear thinking, and nursing research courses as a way to study—for many years. Increasingly, students are more accepting of them as a way to learn but we still have students who balk at them. They want linear formats—columns and outlines—because that's what they've used for years. But, for others it has become very liberating as their brains can now focus more naturally on the whole along with the parts in a matrix pattern instead of straight lines.

From Constant Success to Failure Possibilities

If you are going to be innovative, you must risk failure and that's that. Now, think about that in today's society that values success over all else, and you'll see the difficulties in moving toward this kind of thinking. While we were writing this, there was a news item about physicist Stephen Hawking admitting that he was wrong about black holes (Pogatchnik, 2004). He has now revised his theory that has been considered flawless since the 1980s. It was great to see that news item, not because he failed, but because he was so matter-of-fact about his "failure." He exhibited *intellectual integrity*. Great ideas don't just appear wrapped up neatly; they develop over time with experimentation and repeated failures preceding their success. This is another area where Senge (1998) is adamant—innovation is a process of failure, and true learning doesn't occur when we train

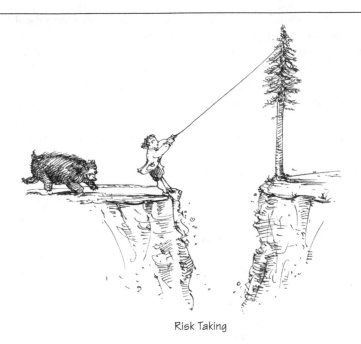

Risk Taking

people to avoid failure. There's a story about Thomas Edison who, in response to a reporter who asked about his failed results while inventing the lightbulb, replied, "Results? Why, man, I have gotten lots of results! If I find 10,000 ways something won't work, I haven't failed. I am not discouraged, because every wrong attempt discarded is often a step forward" (Beals, 1996).

From Valuing Only Objectivity to Being Open to Intuition

You'll note that we have a qualifying adjective there—"only"; we don't want to imply that we shouldn't value objectivity, but we have to be careful that we don't ignore intuition in our attempts to overcome bias and be objective. As you know by now, *intuition* was identified and defined in our consensus research on CT in nursing (Scheffer & Rubenfeld, 2000) as "insightful sense of knowing without conscious use of reason" (p. 358). Polanyi (1964) described it years ago as "tacit knowing." It has been studied extensively in nursing, the most notable being Benner and Tanner's (1987) work. Effken (2001), after an extensive review of literature, placed *intuition* in an ecological psychology framework, allowing us to look beyond cognitive or perceptual processes to ". . . the information provided by the patient and the context of care" (p. 252).

Viewing *intuition* in this way links it with *contextual perspective*, making it valuable in living systems environments. *Intuitive* responses take in a broader view of events and that's what we need today. Rosanoff (1999) saw deeper *intuitive* responses as valuable in today's healthcare world where quick decisions are called for. She suggested tactics to promote *intuition*— stop and look inside for your *intuitive* response, practice being attentive to *intuitive* responses, keep a journal of your *intuitive* responses to see how accurate they are. She even suggested starting meetings by asking members to look at the agenda, record their thoughts and feelings, and then share them. This probably would enhance *intuitive* responses if those directions were couched in *intuitive* sounding words such as "your first gut reactions," "immediate hunches," and so forth. Senge (1996) suggested a similar process of meeting check-ins and check-outs focused on the thinking of participants.

From Reviewing to Reflection

The final pattern of change in thinking needed today is perhaps self-evident. If you have read the preceding pages in one sitting, go back now and review what you read. After you've done that, *reflect* on what you've read. How are reviewing and *reflection* different? Reviewing can be done fairly passively, but *reflection* can't. You have to put your personal self into *reflection* because it's deeper thinking. The Delphi study consensus group defined *reflection* as "contemplation upon a subject, especially one's assumptions and thinking for the purposes of deeper understanding and self-evaluation" (Scheffer & Rubenfeld, 2000, p. 358).

That deeper understanding and self-evaluation is where you need to be to prepare for the challenges of today's and tomorrow's healthcare delivery and education. The old thinking will not work; you need to evaluate yourself and your present thinking patterns and contemplate what you need to do to transform them to meet present and future needs.

At this point, we'd like to share with you a nurse's story. While she doesn't describe her thinking that much, it's quite easy to see how her thinking fits with the moves we have described above. What do you think?

HOW ONE NURSE'S THINKING HELPED HER MEET THE 5 IOM COMPETENCIES

Marcia Hegstad is a Clinical Nurse Specialist for Diabetes at a large teaching hospital in Michigan. We mentioned her briefly in Chapter 8. She is the epitome of a nurse demonstrating all five of the IOM competencies. She wouldn't describe it in those terms but it is easy to see "patient-centered care," "working in interdisciplinary teams," "using evidence-based practice," "using informatics," and "improving quality" in her story. She is very matter-of-fact in reporting this great work; we get the feeling she sees it as "normal" patient care, but we were gleeful hearing a report of such excellence. After you read her story we'll look at her thinking. Here she discusses a project to use the best evidence in glycemic control with diabetics undergoing cardiac surgery (personal communication, Marcia Hegstad, July 20, 2004):

I started this somewhere around 1997 for two reasons. I was asked by the heart surgeons to assist in the management of blood glucose of several patients close together. We had several post cardiac surgery patients readmitted to the ICU with deep sternal wound infections. I noticed in the literature that there were reports of the relationship between hyperglycemia and post-op infections. It really bothered me and I decided to look at some charts and saw that these patients had hyperglycemia pre-operatively.

Around the same time I got a call from a graduate student who was interested in doing a thesis about controlling infections in heart patients. I told her it was "weird" that she had called me because I had just been looking at this. She told me about an article by Zerr and Furnary in the Annals of Thoracic Surgery *(Zerr, Furnary, Grunkemeier, Bookin, Kanhere, & Starr, 1997) that had compelling information about a definite relationship between pre-op hyperglycemia and deep sternal infections. These authors had reduced their patients to a less than 200 glucose for the first 3 days post-op and had decreased infections.*

I did a retrospective chart audit and saw that the patients with infections had glucose readings above 200. I went to the cardio-thoracic surgeons who said they didn't like the infections either and they wanted to do something about this. I told them about the article. We teamed up the endocrinology, SICU and step-down staff and developed protocols for post-op insulin drips. Then we talked to an anesthesiologist about this. We called Anthony Furnary who said he moved the insulin drips into the OR and had essentially eradicated these infections. The anesthesiologist's eyes nearly popped out of his head and we moved it to the OR. We targeted glucose at 200 and patients did very well. We had months with no deep sternal infections.

I was able to track these data through the Infection Control Department which has a tracking system for infections so getting the data was pretty simple. The Anesthesiology Department looked at records with me and could see the patterns.

When we started this project there wasn't much evidence except to keep glucose below 200. Furnary is now keeping patients between 100 and 150 instead of 200. (See Furnary et al., 2003.) Less than 200 was good for preventing deep sternal infections but he reported that superficial infections are also controlled with even lower glucoses. We keep them between 125 and 175 now. We'll probably move to keeping them even lower but we have to remem-

ber that, during surgery, we have direct technology to see blood pressure, heart rate, etc. on a monitor but we have to do more to monitor blood sugar and we have to be sensitive to this technology issue.

This has been an endless process of encouraging, monitoring, giving feed-back and so forth. There are so many people involved, such as endocrinolo-gists, physician assistants, surgeons, anesthesiologists, OR perfusionists, and nurses in ICU and step-down units. It has been great interdisciplinary team-work. This work has been picked up by another hospital; I'm not sure they're using the protocols just as we developed them or if they've adapted them.

This is obviously a condensed version of these years of work, eliminating numerous meetings with diverse teams of providers, gathering information, dis-cussions, trials, revisions, and so forth. She used the best available evidence but, because it was still scarce at the start of the project, the team proceeded with caution. As the evidence grew, so did their plan. (See, for example, Zerr et al., 1997; Furnary, Zerr, Grunkemeier, & Starr, 1999; Furnary et al., 2003; Clement et al., 2004). Her use of the available informatics in tracking data al-lowed her and her team to see patterns. This endeavor, initiated by a nurse who was concerned about patients' conditions enough to launch a huge change of practice, resulted in significant quality improvement. We think the IOM team should salute her for illustrating what they are trying to get others to achieve.

Look at the hints to Marcia's thinking in this story and compare them to the patterns of change we've been discussing. She certainly was engaged; she focused on questions, not just answers, and combined thinking and doing. She admits this project is not yet completed—a journey, not a destination. She was proactive in her learning—no one told her to do this. She acknowledged the complexities of her system. There certainly were few dichotomous statements; she was looking at a whole, not just pieces. She clearly did her thinking with others, not just on her own. There were no attempts to gloss over the complexities. She saw new pat-terns and did not take a linear approach to the project. The project has taken sev-eral years, so we doubt that every step along the way has been without failures. Marcia's beginning statements imply an *intuitive* response as she questioned practice. She clearly has *reflected* on this and, if you could have heard her talk, as we did, you'd know *intuitively* that she is a constantly *reflective*, humble person.

PAUSE AND PONDER:
THE HARD WORK OF THINKING

If we thought yesterday's thinking was hard, based on today's thinking we can project tomorrow's thinking to be even harder. Do you think that's true? Certainly the context is getting more and more complex. However, it could get easier. Remember when we tried to use CT in the context of yesteday's view of systems as mechanistic and it didn't fit? CT fits better with systems that are nonlinear and dynamic—complex adaptive systems. Today critical thinkers are still considered troublemakers in some systems; however, that is changing, and clinicians and educators with CT abilities are gaining acceptance and are being held up as people who have superior survival skills. If you're sitting there saying we've gone a bit wifty again, you might want to reconsider because we think we're on track and there are many who seem to agree.

Reflection Cues

- This chapter is the second "bookend" chapter, along with Chapter 5, that encloses the five chapters on CT and the IOM competencies.
- The overwhelming message in discussions of the five competencies is change—change in healthcare delivery and education.
- New conceptualizations of change are needed for today's complex world.
- Realistic models for change in healthcare and education come from living, adaptive systems, not the older mechanistic models.
- Today's systems are dynamically complex, so that change is constant and each part of the system that changes influences all other parts of the system.
- Old thinking patterns will not work with the reality of today and the near future.
- Fifteen patterns of change in thinking are described: passivity to engagement; answers to questions; separate thinking and doing to thinking and doing together; destination to journey; reactive to proactive learning; mechanistic to living system models; dichotomous to relativistic thinking; pieces to wholes; alone to systems; reduction to complexity; matching existing patterns to new patterns; linear to maps/knots/shapes; constant success to failure possibilities; valuing only objectivity to being open to *intuition*; and reviewing to *reflecting*.
- One nurse's story of changing care of surgical patients with diabetes illustrates the five IOM competencies and new patterns of thinking.
- Critical thinkers will fit better with systems that are complex and adaptive.

References

Beals, G. (1996). Thomas Edison "Quotes." Retrieved August 10, 2004, from http://www.thomasedison.com/edquote.htm.

Benner, P. & Tanner, C. (1987). Clinical judgment: How expert nurses use intuition. *American Journal of Nursing, 87,* 23–31.

Clement, S., Braithwaite, S. S., Magee, M. F., Ahmann, A., Smith, E. P., Schafer, R. G., & Hirsch, I. B. (2004). Management of diabetes and hyperglycemia in hospitals. *Diabetes Care, 27*(2), 553–591.

Effken, J. A. (2001). Informational basis for expert intuition. *Journal of Advanced Nursing, 34*(2), 246–255.

Estabrooks, C. A. (2003). Translating research into practice: Implications for organizations and administrators. *Canadian Journal of Nursing Research, 35*(3), 53–68.

Fullan, M. (1993). *Change forces: Probing the depths of educational reform.* Briston, PA: The Falmer Press.

Furnary, A. P., Zerr, K. J., Grunkemeier, G. L., & Starr, A. (1999). Continuous intravenous insulin infusion reduces the incidence of deep sternal wound infection in diabetic patients after cardiac surgical procedures. *Annals of Thoracic Surgery, 67*, 352–362.

Furnary, A. P., Gao, G., Grunkemeier, G. L., Wu, X. X., Zerr, K. J., Bookin, S. O., Floten, H. S., & Starr, A. (2003). Continuous insulin infusion reduces mortality in patients with diabetes undergoing coronary artery bypass grafting. *The Journal of Thoracic and Cardiovascular Surgery, 125*, 1007–1021.

Hart, L. A. (1983). *Human brain and human learning.* New York: Longman.

Institute of Medicine. (2003). *Health professions education: A bridge to quality.* Washington, DC: National Academies Press.

Mueller, A., Johnston, M., & Bligh, D. (2002). Joining mind mapping and care planning to enhance student critical thinking and achieve holistic nursing care. *Nursing Diagnosis, 13*(1), 24–27.

Novak, J. D. (1998). *Learning, creating, and using knowledge: Concept maps as facilitative tools in schools and corporations.* Mahwah, NJ: Lawrence Erlbaum Associates.

Perkins, D. N. (1994). *The intelligent eye: Learning to think by looking at art.* Los Angeles: J. Paul Getty Trust.

Plsek, P. (2003, January). *Complexity and the Adoption of Innovation in Health Care.* Paper presented at the conference *Accelerating Quality Improvement in Health Care Strategies to Speed the Diffusion of Evidence-based Innovations,* by National Institute for Health Care Management Foundation and National Committee for Quality Health Care, Washington, DC.

Plsek, P. E. & Greenhalgh, T. (2001). The challenge of complexity in health care. *BMJ, 323,* 625–628. Retrieved July 21, 2004, from http://bmj.bmjjournals.com/cgi/content/full/323/7313/625.

Pogatchnik, S. (2004, July 22). *Physicist's black holes theory turns inside out.* Associated Press as reported in *The Detroit Free Press,* Thursday, July 22, 2004.

Polanyi, M. (1964). The logic of tacit inference. In Grene, M. (Ed.). *Knowing and Being: Essays by Michael Polanyi* (pp. 138–158). Chicago: University of Chicago Press.

Porter-O'Grady, T. (2003). Innovation and creativity in a new age for health care. *Journal of the New York State Nurses Association, 34*(2), 4–8.

Rideout, E. (2001). *Transforming nursing education through problem-based learning.* Boston: Jones and Bartlett.

Rosanoff, N. (1999). Intuition comes of age: Workplace applications of intuitive skill for occupational and environmental health nurses. *AAOHN Journal, 47*(4), 156–162.

Scheffer, B. K. & Rubenfeld, M. G. (2000). A consensus statement on critical thinking in nursing. *Journal of Nursing Education, 39*(8), 352–359.

Senge, P. M. (1990). *The fifth discipline: The art & practice of the learning organization.* New York: Doubleday.

Senge, P. M. (1996, Fall). The ecology of leadership. *Leader to Leader, 2*, 18–23. Retrieved July 21, 2004, from http://www.pfdf.org/leaderbooks/L2L/fall96/senge.html.

Senge, P. M. (1998, 2004). *Leadership in the world of the living* (An essay from *The Dance of Change*). Washington, DC: The Center for Association Leadership. Retrieved July 21, 2004, from http://www.gwsae.org/ThoughtLeaders/SengeLeadership.htm.

Senge P. M. (1998, Summer). The practice of innovation. *Leader to Leader, 9*, 16–22. Retrieved July 21, 2004, from http://www.pdf.org/leaderbooks/L2L/summer98/senge.html.

Senge, P. M., Scharmer, C. O., Jaworski, J., & Flowers, B. S. (2004). Awakening faith in an alternative future. *Reflections: The Society for Organizational Learning Journal on Knowledge, Learning, and Change, 5*(7), 1–11. Retrieved July 21, 2004, from: http://www.reflections.solonline.org.

Waldman, J. D., Smith, H. L., & Hood, J. N. (2003). Corporate culture: The missing piece of the healthcare puzzle. *Hospital Topics, 81*(1), 5–14.

Wheeler, L. A. & Collins, S. K. R. (2003). The influence of concept mapping on critical thinking in baccalaureate nursing students. *Journal of Professional Nursing, 19*(96), 339–346.

Zerr, K. J., Furnary, A. P., Grunkemeier, G. L., Bookin, S., Kanhere, V., & Starr, A. (1997). Glucose control lowers the risk of wound infection in diabetics after open heart operations. *Annals of Thoracic Surgery, 63*, 356–361.

CHAPTER 12

Assessing Critical Thinking

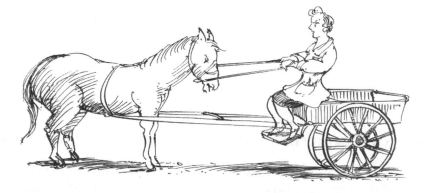

We have left this chapter until last for several reasons. First and foremost, we wanted to say all those things about critical thinking—what it is, how complex it is, how the dynamic context of healthcare affects and is affected by CT, how it fits with current desired competencies in healthcare, and how it plays out in real life—before we discussed how it might be evaluated. We believe the present approach to evaluation has imposed a very reductionist view of CT in nursing; educators and clinicians have been led to believe CT can be put into boxes to be dichotomously checked off. They have been using instruments that have little validity for nursing because they weren't based on descriptions of CT in nursing.

Second, we believe nurses, especially in nursing education, jumped on the bandwagon of evaluating CT in the early 1990s, largely in response to accreditation standards, before they really understood what CT was all about. They started evaluating something that they probably weren't overtly teaching. At the very least there was incongruence between what was being taught and what was being assessed. We want to make sure the horse gets in front of the cart and not the other way around.

These issues—CT complexity and pressures to evaluate CT—are interrelated. Quantitative measuring instruments cannot capture the complexity of CT, but they are popular because of their ease of use. Qualitative processes can capture the complexity, but they are cumbersome and require more resources to use. Outside pressures to measure CT have pushed educators to find measurement instruments quickly. No objective measures so far accurately reflect what anecdotal reports from clinicians and educators show. Finding a suitable measure has been the most difficult problem in meeting the critical thinking accreditation criterion (Stone, Davidson, Evans, & Hansen, 2001).

Finally (third), we want you to have a stage from which you can view our suggestions for CT evaluation processes—one with a real-life view of CT. After completing the research to find a consensus on CT in nursing, we found that while there were many similarities between our statement and other definitions of CT, there were also unique components. Whether these are unique to nursing or characteristic of healthcare disciplines or applied sciences remains to be seen. (You may want to review Chapter 2 to see *what* we're talking about relative to those unique areas of CT.) Because we've become convinced that CT in nursing has some discipline-specific characteristics, we don't believe it can adequately be assessed with non-nursing instruments.

CLARIFICATION OF THE WORDS *ASSESSMENT* AND *EVALUATION*

Before we launch into details of these topics we'd like to discuss why we've used the word "assessment" instead of "evaluation" in our title and why we're going to switch to its use from here on. First of all, what we call "evaluation" in nursing is often referred to as "assessment" in other fields—education and business in particular. "Evaluation" has a connotation of right or wrong; "assessment" implies data collection or measurement followed by interpretation, but the interpretation is not necessarily a judgment of right or wrong.

The nursing profession may have gone over to the word "evaluation" because of the established description of the nursing process, where "assessment" means collecting data and interpreting patients' needs, and "evaluation" means determining if the patient has met the goals outlined in our plans of care after the implementation of planned interventions. In reality, our nursing process "evaluation" is another "assessment" with goals as a standard of comparison.

CT is not a right or wrong thing—it just is. Everyone thinks; granted some do it better and more critically than others, but we rarely come to conclusions that someone's totality of thinking was wrong. Because most healthcare professionals are still discussing what CT actually is, we're a long way from being able to say that this thinking is right and that thinking is wrong. Most people would be hard-pressed to even say how one person's thinking is better than another's.

OK, can we live with "assessment" being the better word for now? We'll assume you all nodded your heads, so we'll move on to a discussion of the points we laid out in the introduction to this chapter.

THE RELEVANCE OF CT COMPLEXITY TO ASSESSMENT OF CT

Whew! That subtitle alone is complex, isn't it? How do you assess something complex? First of all you need to articulate what that complex phenomenon is. Then you must break it down into understandable parts without losing track of the whole. As you have probably figured out by now, that's no easy task with CT. We've given you a complex set of 17 dimensions that an international panel of nurses arrived at through a long process of consensus (Scheffer & Rubenfeld, 2000). That research-based description is only now starting to be cited in nursing literature and to be used by clinicians, researchers, and educators (e.g., Ali, Bantz, & Siktberg, 2005; Allen, Rubenfeld, & Scheffer, 2004; Lunney, 2003; Staib, 2003; Tanner, 2005; Twibell, Ryan, & Hermiz, 2005).

If we accept the complexity of CT in nursing, what does this mean in terms of assessing CT of clinicians and students? Assessment instruments, to have any validity, must measure what they purport to measure. (Remember Research 101!) Multiple-choice tests are very popular because they provide "objective" numerical data that can be analyzed in varying configurations to show results for individuals and groups. They can be used easily, requiring very few personnel resources, and are, therefore, very desirable in fields such as nursing, which require lots of resources anyway. However, measuring something as complex as CT via quantitative measures is very difficult; items have to be cleaned up enough so that the instrument has reliability, and in that process of "clean up" it is easy to lose what is important. In the process of reducing a complex concept to reach reliability, validity can very easily go out the window.

There has been little consistency to the definitions of CT used by nursing over the years; descriptions are as varied as nursing programs (Scheffer, 2001). Nevertheless, educators have been assessing CT with standardized multiple-choice tests for quite some time. However, the CT tests most commonly used are not based on descriptions of nursing CT; rather they are based on more general descriptions of CT. Unfortunately these tests, according to the nursing literature, show little increase in students' CT ability while in school (Adams, 1999; Staib, 2003). The need for discipline-specific CT instruments has been addressed repeatedly (e.g., Allen, Rubenfeld, & Scheffer, 2004; Beckie, Lowry, & Barnett, 2001; Stone et al., 2001).

There are many reasons postulated for the inability to show objectively that students learn CT while in nursing school, the major one being that these tests lack validity for nursing because they are not based on definitions of CT in the field. For a concise review of these commonly used multiple-choice instruments, see Staib (2003): Watson-Glaser Critical Thinking Appraisal, California Critical Thinking Skills Test, California Critical Thinking Dispositions Inventory, Minnesota Test of Critical Thinking. The National League for Nursing (2004) developed a nursing-based multiple-choice CT instrument but, because it is new, research on its effectiveness to show CT change is unavailable.

When we conduct workshops on CT around the world, we are frequently asked questions about CT assessment instruments. Academic-based educators are particularly frustrated with their present instruments. Practice-based educators haven't been using these instruments but are interested in how they can assess CT in their staff. Clinicians want to know how they can see if their CT is on track.

THE CART BEFORE THE HORSE PROBLEM WITH ASSESSING CT

"Incomplete or premature assessment destroys learning" (Senge, 1998, np, 4th section, para 2). This should probably be posted in meeting rooms as academic-based educators contemplate accreditation visits and should appear in front of clinicians who look around at their colleagues and conclude there is little CT going on. In the same section of the document cited above, Senge quoted Bill O'Brien, retired CEO of Hanover Insurance, as saying "managers are always pulling up the radishes to see how they're growing."

This is what we've been doing—pulling up the radishes, a.k.a., premature assessment. Some of the push for CT assessment has come from accrediting bodies. The National League for Nursing Accrediting Commission (NLN-AC) (2000) and the Commission on Collegiate Nursing Education (CCNE) (2003) both value CT and ask directly (NLN-AC) or indirectly (CCNE) for evidence of

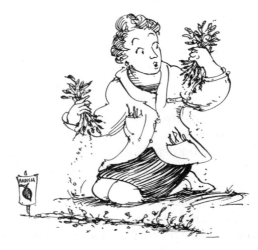

CT in nursing curricula. CCNE asks that *The Essentials of Baccalaureate Education for Professional Nursing Practice* (AACN, 1998) be used to guide programs; that document lists CT as part of the expected core competencies.

We started, at least in academic settings, assessing CT before we articulated what it was, how best to teach it, and, indeed, whether we were teaching it at all. We valued CT and we've been quite sure that nurses use CT. However, we mistook our valuing of the idea and assumptions about CT; we thought that meant we were teaching it; we thought students were learning it. In reality, we were assessing things that we didn't understand well, had difficulty articulating, and probably were not teaching.

Figure 12.1 is something we've used in workshops with academic-based educators who struggle to link CT with assessment. It's a simple idea, but one easily overlooked. We ask educators to look at their expected program outcomes and follow the various steps along the way toward evaluation mechanisms; the steps in between are theoretical and operational definitions of CT, course objectives, CT course content and teaching strategies, and finally, evaluation. Educators often express surprise when they see they have gaps or inconsistencies

Figure 12.1   Consistency of CT in Academic Programs

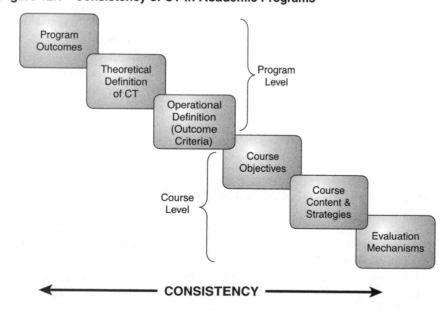

in that sequence; they have course objectives related to CT, but no real definition of it, for example. Often, they have CT in the "evaluation mechanisms" box, but nowhere else. They know it is important and accreditors are looking for it. CT is "tacked on" instead of being integrated into programs.

We see the same "tacking on" happening in textbooks. CT exercises have become the norm in most of the big undergraduate texts for adult health, obstetrical, pediatric, community health nursing, and so forth. However, if you look closely at many of those texts, you might wonder why those particular exercises are characterized as CT and how the authors are defining CT. There is often an assumption that everyone knows what it is and everyone defines it the same way. In reality, if you ask many faculty how they are defining CT in their programs, they will have trouble answering (Scheffer, 2001).

There is some danger that clinicians will be subjected to the same faulty means of assessment that have occurred in academic settings as, increasingly, there are messages that nurses must be good critical thinkers to promote safety, increase quality, and so on. Administrators and managers will look for quick assessment instruments to give a numerical thinking number to nurses. We are sometimes asked if we have remedial CT courses for nurses who have made serious mistakes and who need to improve their thinking. (We don't.) That kind of simplistic approach to CT makes it seem like any other tacked-on skill that can be fixed with a refresher course.

Because of our concerns about making the same mistakes in practice settings as in academic settings, we have included Figure 12.2, which shows organizational tracking points when looking for consistency in CT. If personnel in practice settings value CT enough to evaluate it, they must be careful to consistently define it in mission statements, aims, objectives, expectations, and so forth.

CT must be integrated throughout clinical and educational programs. All the other things we teach, learn, and practice provide the context for CT. It can't be separated or tacked on. It must be defined, described, taught, and practiced. Clinicians and learners must have time to describe their thinking, practice it, and demonstrate it before being assessed on how they've learned it. Assessment of CT must be linked to expectations and behaviors.

LINKING TEACHING, LEARNING, AND PRACTICING CT WITH ASSESSMENT OF CT

If we accept that healthcare delivery and education occur in complex, adaptive, learning environments, then we want to make sure that we assess what is being learned using methods that address complexity and are also adaptive. Trying to take the complexity out of CT for the purpose of having clean, quantitative tools won't provide a picture of how we, and the people around us, are doing

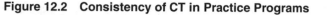

Figure 12.2   Consistency of CT in Practice Programs

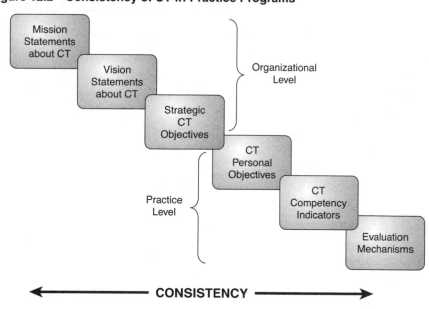

with CT. Neither will we get a picture of CT if our assessment procedures are so vague that no one understands what is being assessed. In Box 12.1 we have outlined some considerations for your journey toward valid assessment of CT.

First, have a clear idea of what CT is for your organization. Is it defined as a complex collection of cognitive skills and affective habits of the mind, or is it overly simplified? Beware if it's defined very simply. The definition may have been driven by the assessment method—defined after the fact to fit with an instrument. That's the tail wagging the dog. If there's no description to be found anywhere, then consider if you need one. Is CT important in your organization? It should be in today's complex healthcare delivery and education. You may be the person who needs to develop, adopt, or adapt a description of your organization's thinking model.

If you find a very complex description of CT, is it broken down into manageable components or presented as an operational definition so that it could be assessed? If it hasn't been, then beware because chances are CT is not being assessed, or there is a misfit between the definition and the assessment process.

If there is no assessment plan in place, should there be one? If your answer is yes, then, as with finding a description, it may be up to you to develop,

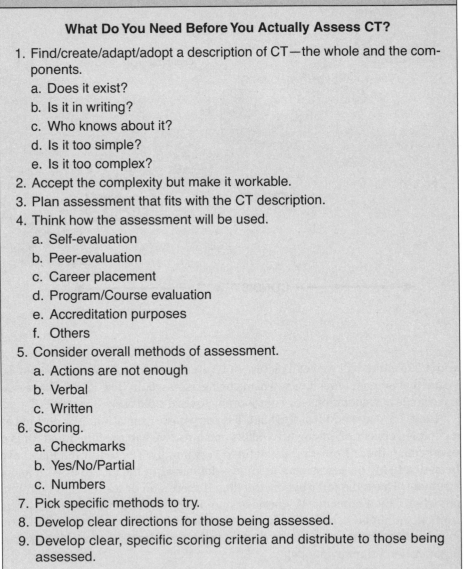

Box 12.1

What Do You Need Before You Actually Assess CT?

1. Find/create/adapt/adopt a description of CT—the whole and the components.
   a. Does it exist?
   b. Is it in writing?
   c. Who knows about it?
   d. Is it too simple?
   e. Is it too complex?
2. Accept the complexity but make it workable.
3. Plan assessment that fits with the CT description.
4. Think how the assessment will be used.
   a. Self-evaluation
   b. Peer-evaluation
   c. Career placement
   d. Program/Course evaluation
   e. Accreditation purposes
   f. Others
5. Consider overall methods of assessment.
   a. Actions are not enough
   b. Verbal
   c. Written
6. Scoring.
   a. Checkmarks
   b. Yes/No/Partial
   c. Numbers
7. Pick specific methods to try.
8. Develop clear directions for those being assessed.
9. Develop clear, specific scoring criteria and distribute to those being assessed.

adapt, or adopt one. If there is a description and an operational, working model of CT, then you can make a list of what should be assessed. Now you have to consider what the assessment results will be used for. Will they be for staff performance evaluations? Self-evaluations? Peer evaluations? Career advancement? Program evaluation? Course grades? Accreditation justification? Obviously, those questions and answers will be largely institutional-specific.

Once you have those answers, then you're ready to consider various methods of assessment. We have some suggestions, but first we'd like to address a question that often emerges at this point. Maybe you haven't considered this, but many nurses ask, "Isn't what I do (or my students or staff do) proof enough of CT, that is, isn't it all about actions anyway?" The answer to that is, it depends. Sometimes actions can show CT; sometimes not. You might see the same actions from two people, but the first one just happened to see the second one doing something and mimicked the behavior. The second one might have spent hours of thinking to come up with that approach. It's only when you start asking them to describe why they're doing what they're doing that you begin to see the thinking. The mimic will likely have trouble adapting the action to a different set of circumstances because the background thinking hasn't occurred.

To assess thinking, we need the person's descriptions of his/her thinking to judge that thinking. In Chapter 2 we described the necessity of a thinking vocabulary to understand CT (see Box 2.5). We also need it to assess CT.

So, you either need to hear or read a person's description of thinking to assess that thinking. Now comes the harder part. How can you do that in ways that will meet all of your needs? Does it always have to be set up like an interview or an essay? No. Do you have to spend hours reading and/or listening to these "answers" to make a judgment about how someone is thinking? No. Can you ever get numerical data from such seemingly qualitative assessment processes? Yes.

Much of the challenge in these assessment methods is setting up the criteria for judging quality. We're so conditioned to the right or wrong mentality that is implicit in multiple-choice questions that it's hard to see alternatives. First, be very clear in your directions for assignments used to assess CT. If the directions are fuzzy, the person being assessed will waste valuable thinking time trying to figure out what is expected. Next, set up the "scoring" ahead of time and tell the person how s/he is being assessed. Is it going to be a yes (that thinking dimension was demonstrated) or no (the dimension was not demonstrated)? Will there be a middle ground (the dimension was partially demonstrated)? Will you assign numbers or letters to those criteria? Remember, in order to set up specific criteria, you, as the assessor, must know what you are assessing. Once again, you must know what CT is and how you and your organization define it and its parameters.

In the next two sections of this chapter, we will provide suggestions of practical methods to assess CT. In the first section we will report briefly on our latest research, where we studied a quantitative approach. We assessed all dimensions of CT, assigned numbers, and checked out the reliability of that method. In the final section we have descriptions of methods we have used in workshops and classes for which we have only anecdotal evidence of their success.

ONE SUGGESTION FOR A REALISTIC QUANTITATIVE METHOD TO ASSESS CT IN NURSING WITHOUT LOSING CT'S COMPLEXITY

As soon as we finished the Delphi study to find a consensus on CT in nursing, people started asking us if we had an instrument based on that description of CT. Initially we raised our fingers in front of us, crossed them and said, "No way are we doing psychometric research!!" Most of you probably understand our aversion to the long process of developing an instrument. In addition, the more we studied CT, the more we realized that an objective, multiple-choice-type test could never test all dimensions of CT. We also realized that essay-type tests such as the Ennis-Weir Critical Thinking Essay Test (Ennis & Weir, 1985) would be very time-consuming and not helpful to tracking aggregate data.

In our courses, we started assigning students *reflection* assignments to show their CT and to help them learn the vocabulary necessary to articulate their abstract thinking processes. Sometimes we gave them vignettes and asked them to do something to show their thinking. At other times, especially in clinical courses, we asked them to reflect on events from their clinical time to show their thinking. We used the 17 dimensions of CT from our research to give direction so students could zero in on specific parts of the thinking processes. They wrote about one or two dimensions at a time, not all 17. Over the course of a semester or year, they addressed all dimensions of CT.

As any educator will tell you, grading essays can be extremely time-consuming. To save ourselves time, we developed scoring rubrics to give to students ahead of time so they would know what a 3 or a 2 meant. Then we could just put numerical scores on their papers. After we tried this for a couple years, we considered that it might work as a more formal means of assessing CT. We knew that, because we were basing this work on a research-derived description of CT in nursing, we had some validity going for us. However, we weren't sure if our assessment procedure could be done reliably by others. We decided it was time for help from someone more knowledgeable about psychometrics and statistics than we were. Enter Dr. George Allen from Michigan State University, "up the road" from us at Eastern Michigan University. We teamed up with George and told him about our consideration of reflection assignments graded with a scoring rubric as a means to reliably assess CT in nursing students.

We developed a plan and piloted it at four schools with undergraduate nursing students. Because we knew that assessment must be linked with teaching and learning we conducted workshops for those faculty and described the procedure for assessment. The faculty who agreed to try this in a course assigned the *reflections*, scored them using the rubric, sent them to George, who sent them blind to the two of us. We scored them independently, sent them back to George, who analyzed the results for reliability. We were happy to see that our coefficient alphas

Box 12.2

Examples of Methods of Tracking CT Dimensions

Example #1:

Compiling <u>Individual</u> Student Data on CT Skills and Habits of the Mind

Student Name_____ ID#_____

Undergraduate____   Graduate____

<u>Dimension</u>   <u>Scores</u>

Course____   Course____   Course____

	Course	Course	Course
Confidence	_____	_____	_____
Contextual Perspective	_____	_____	_____
Creativity	_____	_____	_____
Flexibility	_____	_____	_____

(and so forth for all dimensions)

Example #2:

Aggregate <u>Course</u> Data on Critical Thinking Skills and Habits of the Mind

Undergraduate____   Graduate____   Semester/Year____

Averages of Scores for All Students

Course____   Course____   Course____

	Course	Course	Course
# of Students	_____	_____	_____
<u>Dimensions:</u>			
Confidence	_____	_____	_____
Contextual Perspective	_____	_____	_____
Creativity	_____	_____	_____

(and so forth for all dimensions)

Example #3:

Aggregate <u>Entry/Exit</u> Year Data on Critical Thinking Skills and Habits of the Mind

Undergraduate____   Graduate____

	Year____	Year____
# of Students	_____	_____
Dimensions: Average Scores for All Students in Year		
Confidence	_____	_____
Contextual Perspective	_____	_____
Creativity	_____	_____
Flexibility	_____	_____

(and so forth for all dimensions)

for inter-rater reliability were between 0.70 and 0.80, which, for educational purposes, according to most authorities is quite satisfactory (e.g., Nunnally, 2002). For a detailed report of this research, see Allen, Rubenfeld, & Scheffer (2004).

We learned from this process that short essay-type CT reflection assignments may be scored quite quickly using a rubric. It took us between 1 to 2 minutes to score each assignment after doing the first few. Remember, we weren't grading things like grammar and writing style, so we did not have to insert written comments as we read; we just used the rubric and assigned numbers. We need to keep that in mind; nursing faculty often feel the need to grade all written projects for writing style. If that is your aim, do it with other assignments, not those where you primarily want to assess CT. If you want a numerical assessment of CT so you can track aggregate data, then using scoring rubrics allows you to maintain the complexity of CT, but in a simple tool. Box 12.2 provides several examples of such tracking forms.

OTHER SPECIFIC TACTICS FOR ASSESSING CT

In Box 12.3 are several methods that can be used to assess CT. List A includes strategies to assess all or selected dimensions of CT. List B contains strategies that fit better with some dimensions than with others. In keeping with our view that assessment must be closely linked with teaching, learning, and practicing CT, all these methods may be used both for teaching, learning, and/or assessment purposes.

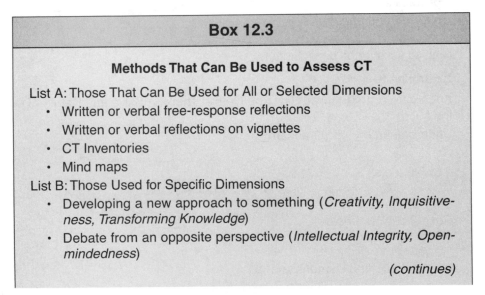

Box 12.3

Methods That Can Be Used to Assess CT

List A: Those That Can Be Used for All or Selected Dimensions
- Written or verbal free-response reflections
- Written or verbal reflections on vignettes
- CT Inventories
- Mind maps

List B: Those Used for Specific Dimensions
- Developing a new approach to something (*Creativity, Inquisitiveness, Transforming Knowledge*)
- Debate from an opposite perspective (*Intellectual Integrity, Open-mindedness*)

(continues)

> ## Box 12.3 *(continued)*
>
> - Differential Diagnosing (*Discriminating, Logical Reasoning, Confidence, Contextual Perspective, Intellectual Integrity, Intuition*)
> - Listing Hunches (*Intuition*)
> - Answering "But, what if..." questions (*Transforming Knowledge, Flexibility*)
> - What is likely to happen to this patient? (*Predicting, Contextual Perspective*)
> - What would you assess next? (*Information Seeking, Discriminating, Contextual Perspective*)
> - What is the principle? (*Applying Standards*)
> - Calling the physician (*Discriminating, Analyzing, Contextual Perspective*)
> - What's wrong with this picture? (*Discriminating*)
> - Critique of literature (*Applying Standards, Discriminating, Analyzing, Logical Reasoning*)
> - Moral Dilemmas (*Analyzing, Intellectual Integrity, Flexibility*)

Free Responses and Vignettes

The first two—free response reflections and reflections on vignettes—are methods used in the research project reported in the previous section. Both types of reflections are written projects focusing on one or two CT dimensions at a time. In a free response, students are asked to reflect on an activity, such as a clinical encounter, and to describe three things: 1) how they demonstrated one or two of the dimensions, such as *creativity* and *intuition*; 2) justification of why that description represents those dimensions and 3) expansion by projecting how they could use those dimensions better next time. These are scored with three numbers, one for each required part of the response, as shown in Box 12.4.

This scoring could, of course, be adapted to one's environment. If you worked with one group of students, all of whom were at the same level of expertise, the third part of the score could be simplified to a 2- or 3-point scale. We used an expertise qualifier so we could show students how their level of knowledge naturally affects their thinking of alternatives and details.

Box 12.5 is an example of a junior student's reflection on a clinical situation where the CT dimension of *flexibility* was used. This was scored as 8; the description clearly identified thinking *flexibility* (2); the student justified this as *flexibility* at the end of the second paragraph (1); and the expansion was very sophisticated—beyond what we'd expect for a second-semester junior (5).

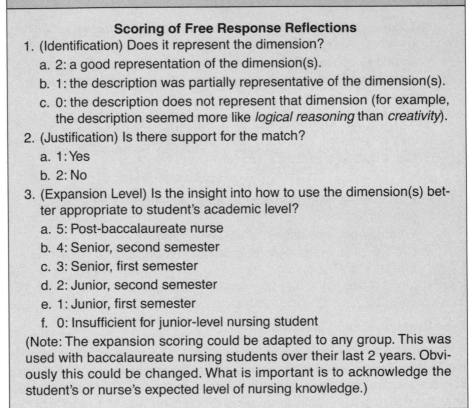

Box 12.4

Scoring of Free Response Reflections

1. (Identification) Does it represent the dimension?
   a. 2: a good representation of the dimension(s).
   b. 1: the description was partially representative of the dimension(s).
   c. 0: the description does not represent that dimension (for example, the description seemed more like *logical reasoning* than *creativity*).
2. (Justification) Is there support for the match?
   a. 1: Yes
   b. 2: No
3. (Expansion Level) Is the insight into how to use the dimension(s) better appropriate to student's academic level?
   a. 5: Post-baccalaureate nurse
   b. 4: Senior, second semester
   c. 3: Senior, first semester
   d. 2: Junior, second semester
   e. 1: Junior, first semester
   f. 0: Insufficient for junior-level nursing student

(Note: The expansion scoring could be adapted to any group. This was used with baccalaureate nursing students over their last 2 years. Obviously this could be changed. What is important is to acknowledge the student's or nurse's expected level of nursing knowledge.)

With vignette responses, students are given a short patient situation/case study and asked to describe how they would do something to demonstrate specified CT dimensions. They are also asked to justify why their description represented those dimensions. These vignette responses are scored with the same scale used for free responses. The expansion (third) part in this case judges the level of detail of the descriptions according to students' class level. Box 12.6 has an example of a vignette assignment.

Obviously, vignettes could be specific to units, levels, or courses. They could be used as a means of assessment (our focus here) or as a teaching/learning focus. Service-based educators could use unit-specific vignettes to help new staff get used to the thinking needed on that unit, for example. Clinicians could write vignettes and prepare a bank of them for others to use.

Box 12.5

Example of a Junior BSN Student Free Response Reflection

One critical thinking reflection dimension that I used during clinical was **flexibility,** the capacity to adapt, accommodate, modify, or change thoughts, ideas, and behaviors. During an interaction with a patient several times I had to adapt my approaches to her. She was bipolar, having psychosis, and was in a severely manic acute phase of the disorder, delusional and hearing voices. In attempting to interact and interview the patient she displayed disorganized and illogical thought processes. She would jump from one topic to the next and even tried to get me to witness her hallucinations. My attempts to obtain information were constantly being hampered and it was difficult to keep her oriented and focused. With every attempt at keeping the patient focused I had to adapt to her various replies. I tried to change my approach and posture in order to find a way to connect with her. When she seemed to be overstimulated by her environment, I moved to the less stimulating atmosphere of the back lounge area. I changed directions in my mind over and over again. I had to appraise the situation and interactions with the patient in my mind.

At first I was at a loss as to how to make the interaction successful. Next, I was overly determined to make it work and even felt frustration starting. Consequently, I thought about stopping and trying again later. Something clicked in my mind that made me realize that silence, a break, and maybe just some time and patience would be beneficial. I realized that maybe my thinking of getting goals accomplished was hampering my thought processes and thus my interviewing abilities. I thought about waiting for a time when her anti-psychotic medication was peaking and then implemented this plan of approach. This approach worked much better and I was able to obtain more information and interact more effectively with my client. Thus, I used **flexibility** in my ability to constantly re-evaluate, adapt, and accommodate to the situation by changing my plan of action.

In this kind of situation again, I'd still need to consider many different alternatives until one worked, but I'd remember from this experience that I always have to be **flexible** in my thinking and actions with these kinds of patients. I would probably not be so fixated on the goals and I'd be less frustrated because I'd turn on my **flexible** thinking right away.

Box 12.6

Example of a Vignette with Student Directions

Directions:

1. Read the clinical vignette below.
2. Read the definition of the critical thinking skill or habit that accompanies the vignette.
3. Describe how you would use the designated critical thinking habit or skill to accomplish the proposed nursing intervention. Include in your description:
   a. What you would do, including enough detail of your thinking to show someone who was not there how you demonstrated the designated habit or skill, and
   b. Why you believe your actions illustrate the designated habit or skill.

(You will be assessed for your ability to accurately represent the critical thinking skill or habit, your justification of how your actions demonstrate the skill or habit, and the specificity of the description.)

Vignette: Charlotte and Mary's Adoption Plans

Critical Thinking Habit of the Mind: ***Intellectual Integrity*** (defined as: *seeking the truth through sincere, honest processes, even if the results are contrary to one's assumptions and beliefs.*)

Charlotte Jones and Mary Kelly are partners who have lived together for 2 years. They are considering adopting a child. They are patients in the obstetrics/gynecology practice where another patient, Susan Simone, is 11 weeks pregnant. Susan is unmarried and wishes to carry her child to term and consider adoption even though her partner, Tom, would rather she had an abortion. Susan, a sophomore in college, is very close to her mother, who is supportive of the plan to offer the child for adoption. Susan has no health insurance and has income only from her part-time job as a waitress. When Susan was told that Charlotte and Mary were interested in adopting her baby, she immediately told the nurse that she wanted to go ahead with whatever was necessary to arrange the adoption.

Describe how you, as the nurse in this situation, would use the *Intellectual Integrity* habit of the mind to help Susan, Charlotte, and Mary **prepare for and interact during their first meeting**.

Both free responses and vignettes can be used as a way to cover all dimensions of CT, but allow for a detailed assessment of each dimension one at a time. These can be used to identify areas of strength and weakness; they allow for individual interpretations, but require that persons be able to justify why they believe their statements represent the particular dimensions. That justification part is important as an overarching logical reasoning. Students must be able to articulate *why* their described thinking logically demonstrates the dimensions. It's not enough to say that they do; such statements must be justified.

Critical Thinking Inventory

The CT Inventory in Appendix A at the back of this book is another method by which to assess all dimensions of CT. This inventory is especially valuable as a self-assessment guide and as a teaching/learning tool to open up minds to the complexities of CT. This is a qualitative approach to assessment; it is difficult to assign numerical points except in terms of clarity, precision, or depth of description. We have used similar instruments for many years, starting with a THINK Inventory in our textbook for beginning level students (Rubenfeld & Scheffer, 1999). It works best for self-evaluation and peer sharing.

Mind Maps

We discussed mind maps in Chapter 5 as an active teaching/learning process, but they can be used to assess CT as well. Most nursing literature on mind mapping or its close cousin, concept mapping, relates to its value in teaching and learning CT (for example, Wheeler & Collins, 2003; Mueller, Johnston, & Bligh, 2002), but there is limited information on their use as an assessment tool. Daley, Shaw, Balistrieri, Glasenapp, & Placentine (1999) outlined a method of assigning points for connecting links in concept maps that had good reliability between two scorers.

ASSESSMENT METHODS FOR SPECIFIC DIMENSIONS OF CT

The remainder of the methods listed in Box 12.3 are useful means of evaluating parts of CT. We'll provide a brief explanation of how these might be used but, as you will see shortly, these methods work best when they are adapted to specific situations.

Developing a new approach to something to show *creativity, inquisitiveness*, and/or *transforming knowledge* may be used to evaluate staff nurses, for example. A career placement assessment could include an innovation criterion. Points could be assigned in accordance with the whole assessment plan when a nurse improves a practice on the unit. This works well with moves toward evidence-based practice (Chapter 8) to reward staff who are innovative in using the best evidence to improve practice.

Debate from an opposite perspective to demonstrate *intellectual integrity* and *open-mindedness* is a valuable exercise for learning and assessment of CT. It is very difficult to debate a controversial issue from a viewpoint opposite your own. Assigning a *reflection* at the end of this exercise can help show the debater's thinking processes. This could be accompanied by a checklist and scored. For example, one could assess the number of issues addressed, the depth of study of those issues, the distance those are from the debater's true beliefs, strength of expression, and so forth.

Differential Diagnosing is a great mechanism to see *discriminating* and *logical reasoning* cognitive skills as well as *confidence, contextual perspective, intellectual integrity,* and *intuition* habits of the mind. Actually a case could be made for using all 17 dimensions in this activity. Using case studies and comparing staff nurses' and clinical experts' diagnosing, Margaret Lunney (2001) reported wide variability in the accuracy of nurses' diagnosing. Lunney (2003) proposed ten CT strategies to promote diagnostic accuracy. A strong case could be made for using her methods and "Scale for Degrees of Accuracy" (2001, p. 36) as a means to assess CT. Making her point especially poignant, Lunney (2003) shared case examples where achieving accuracy of nursing diagnoses was particularly challenging. One was a patient with a T5 fracture who presented with symptoms that the nurse interpreted to be decreased cardiac output; in reality the patient had autonomic dysreflexia. If you look at the signs and symptoms of these two nursing diagnoses (NANDA, 2005, pp. 15 and 26), you can appreciate the necessity of CT to make that distinction.

Listing hunches is related to differential diagnosing as part of the diagnostic process. Taken alone, it can be a good measure of *intuition*. Again, case studies would be used; these could be unit-specific if this method is used by clinicians; they could be class-specific in academic settings. "Experts" in those areas could list their hunches and those lists could be used as a standard for comparison while assessing nurses. Prematurely shutting down one's thinking relative to hunches often leads clinicians to inaccurate conclusions.

Asking and answering "But, what if . . .?" questions is a good way to test for *transforming knowledge* and *flexibility*. At our school, we have been trying this as a component of our skills check-off procedures to add assessment of CT to that process. To use a simple example, think about teaching beginning students to make an occupied bed. Checking their ability to do this merely by watching a demonstration of the classic procedure—turning the patient, pushing the old sheets under him/her, placing new bedding on that side and pushing them under, turning the patient and pulling everything through to the other side and tucking—does little to show you students' thinking. What if you add "But, what if the patient has had a right hip replacement?" That allows you to assess CT. They should, of course, answer with something that indicates they know not to turn the patient on the unaffected hip, therefore internally rotating the replaced hip and causing problems. You want to hear that they can visualize changing the bed from the top of the bed to the bottom or some other plan that maintains hip precautions.

Using case scenarios and asking what is likely to happen to this patient is a method to assess *predicting* and *contextual perspective*. Again, as with many of these assessment examples, this could be made unit-specific if used in practice settings. We often encourage practice-based educators to record case studies for thinking purposes. This is a good thing to have experienced nurses do and, as a way of checking their CT, have them develop the "answers" to whatever questions you'll want to attach to that case study. Then novice nurses can benefit from their collective wisdom. In addition, setting-specific, relevant cases are available for future assessments.

Similar to predicting what is likely to happen to this patient is asking the question, **"What would you assess next?"** This can be used to assess *information seeking*, *discriminating*, and *contextual perspective* dimensions. We have tried this out with RN to BSN students to see what kinds of responses we get. This is a very simple exercise and one that would work well for practice-based educators who want a quick assessment of CT abilities of new nurses. In our trials, we've done this two ways. In the first method, we ask nurses to list the five most important and common patient signs/symptoms found on their units and then to list the parameters they immediately check upon finding those signs/symptoms. In the second method, we give them a list of signs/symptoms and ask them what they think of right away to check. See Box 12.7 for some examples. This exercise could easily be numerically scored using expected assessment standards established by setting-specific experts.

What is the principle? This is a question that promotes *applying standards*. It is also an old assessment technique that was used when we were undergraduates in the 1960s. Asking for standards behind behaviors reveals why someone is doing something and therefore affords the listener a partial picture of that person's thinking. This is an easy assessment method adaptable to almost any setting, quickly separating those who do tasks without much thought and those who know why they are doing something. The latter group is engaged in thinking.

Calling the physician shows *discriminating*, *contextual perspective*, and *analyzing* in particular. It also, incidentally, shows communication skills. This could be applied to calling any other healthcare professional but, because nurses often have to call physicians, this is a familiar situation. Ask physicians about nurse phone calls and they will immediately tell you one of their pet peeves—a nurse who does not seem to have thought through the situation before picking up the phone.

Box 12.7

Sample Answers to the Question, What Would You Assess Next?

Confusion: Check—medications, pulse oximetry, blood pressure, arterial blood gasses, specific neurological signs, temperature, blood glucose, previous mental status patterns, urinalysis, heart rate, headache, weakness

General Complaint of Pain/Discomfort: Check—pain rating, intensity, description, onset, location, duration, history of similar pain, factors that affect, last pain medication time, temperature, pulse oximetry, any surgical/dressing sites

Increased blood pressure: Check—pain, medications, pulse, cardiac rhythm, anxiety, temperature, past history of hypertension, patterns since admission, headache, IV status, recent patient activity; re-check blood pressure manually

Complaint of Constipation: Check—bowel sounds, abdominal distention, tenderness or pain, last bowel movement, how long constipation, past history, links to medical diagnosis, nausea and vomiting, eating pattern, fluid intake, recent GI tests, medications

Decreased Urine Output: Check—intake and output balance, urine color, blood pressure, pulse, temperature, intravenous fluids, weight change, urinalysis, medications such as diuretics, history of renal problems, edema, bladder distention, BUN, creatinine lab values

Request for Darkened Room: Check—depression, headache, history of headaches, fatigue, light sensitivity, privacy issue, drug use

Angry Responses to Staff: Check—what is wrong, pain, fear, anxiety, stress, loss of personal control, family/significant other issue, conflict with specific staff

---

Nurse Smith: "Oh, hi, Dr. Jones; thanks for calling back. Mrs. Frank has only had 100 cc's of urine out in the past 6 hours." Pause. . . . . .

Dr. Jones: "She has heart failure, right?"

Nurse Smith: "Yes, she's been on Lasix."

Dr. Jones: "What was her last dose and when?"

Nurse Smith: "Oh, let me get the med list and check; I just floated down from 700 so I don't know these patients very well."

OK, you get the picture, right? Now, we don't mean to be critical of nurses and being floated to an unfamiliar unit is all too common in the world of hospital-based nurses. Nevertheless, this kind of conversation is very time-consuming and not very helpful because the nurse has not been using much CT.

So, if you were the educator for that unit, you'd probably want to have an in-service on communication and CT. You could use a phone call to a physician as a way of assessing the nurses' level of thinking. Start with a simple situation— Mrs. Frank's urine output has been 100 cc's for 6 hours. Nurse Smith, would you demonstrate your thinking as you prepare for a call to Dr. Jones? Once you do this a few times, you can come up with a list of connections you expect thinking nurses to have made and you'd have your assessment standard.

By the way, you might also invite physicians to your in-service, making it an interdisciplinary session. Communication is a two-way street requiring CT on both sides.

What's wrong with this picture? Asking this question after showing a videotape or presenting a written or verbal case situation is another simple assessment technique that is especially helpful in showing a person's ability to *discriminate*. Our brains are funny things; it is often easier to see when something is wrong than to figure out how to do it right. But, if we can identify what's wrong then we can avoid making that same mistake. Be careful with the "right" or "wrong" messages, though. A better question might be "How can I do this better?"

A critique of literature is a common assessment method used in academic research classes that shows students' abilities to *apply standards, discriminate, analyze,* and *reason logically*. Unfortunately, literature critiques are less commonplace in practice settings. However, as we discussed in Chapter 8, evidence-based practice requires that all clinicians critique articles, guidelines, Internet reports, and so forth. With the indiscriminate glut of information out there, all healthcare providers have to be able to respond critically to that information, and that response requires CT. It is important to know how well those providers can judge the relative merit of that information, so assessing their abilities is becoming more of an issue. Using words like "critique of a report" can be daunting to clinicians who probably see this as an academic exercise, so we recommend you stay away from those words. If you want to assess a person's ability to read something critically, use an article/report that you know has some flaws. (It's harder to find one that doesn't.) Use that article as a measure of CT.

The last suggestion we have in Box 12.2 is to **use moral dilemmas** to assess *analyzing, intellectual integrity,* and *flexibility*. Moving to a relativistic thinking perspective and dealing with the realities of ambiguity in healthcare these days is a vital necessity. There are many moral dilemmas today for which there are no easy answers. How long should we keep a baby alive who has a severe brain problem? Should people over 90 have expensive medical diagnostic tests? How far should we go for stem cell research? Asking someone to respond to a moral dilemma gives important clues to how well they can analyze situations to see the various perspectives, what they are willing to see that might go against conventional answers, and how flexible they are with their possibilities.

PAUSE AND PONDER:
ASSESSMENT IS NOT AN END UNTO ITSELF

There are no simple answers to the challenges in assessing CT. Each approach to judging someone's CT must be scrutinized closely. Remember, this is not something that can be assessed with the same methods we use to assess skills such as giving an injection. CT is not a set of linear steps, but a process that is adapted in various contexts. Because it is complex and dynamic, it calls for assessment methods that are equally dynamic. It is not an end point with specific criteria that can be judged as right or wrong. We must give credit for pieces of CT; for the process, not just the results of thinking. We all have periods when our CT is sharp and periods when it waxes and wanes. Assessment parameters should give credit for the CT waxing and allow for coaching when waning.

Reflection Cues

- Our present approaches to assessing CT in nursing have been reductionistic.
- Nursing education, in particular, has been prone to premature assessment, largely driven by accreditation expectations.
- The complexity of CT does not easily lend itself to simple, quantitative means of assessment.
- The words "evaluation" and "assessment" are often used interchangeably; we have chosen "assessment," which has less of a right-or-wrong connotation.
- Because of CT's complexity, measurement instruments that aim for simplicity and reliability often compromise validity and measure CT incompletely.
- Current methods to assess CT, for the most part, are unable to show the changes in thinking that are reported anecdotally.
- Premature assessment, ahead of clear definitions of CT and consistent operational mechanisms, is problematic.
- Teaching, learning, and practicing CT must be linked with assessment of CT.

- One method to assess CT that maintains complexity, but also allows for quantification; it has been found to have inter-rater reliability.
- Short essays based on free responses and vignettes may be scored reliably with a rubric.
- Various tactics to combine teaching, learning, practicing, and assessing CT are offered.

References

Adams, B. L. (1999). Nursing education for critical thinking: An integrative review. *Journal of Nursing Education, 38*, 111–119.

Ali, N. S., Bantz, D., & Siktberg, L. (2005). Validation of critical thinking skills in online responses. *Journal of Nursing Education, 44*(2), 90–94.

Allen, G. D., Rubenfeld, M. G., & Scheffer, B. K. (2004). Reliability of assessment of critical thinking. *Journal of Professional Nursing, 20*(1), 15–22.

American Association of Colleges of Nursing (1998). *The essentials of baccalaureate education for professional nursing practice.* Washington, DC: Author.

Beckie, T. M., Lowry, L. W., & Barnett, S. (2001). Assessing critical thinking in baccalaureate nursing students: A longitudinal study. *Holistic Nursing Practice, 15*(3), 18–26.

Commission on Collegiate Nursing Education. (2003). *Standards for accreditation of baccalaureate and graduate nursing programs.* Washington, DC: Author.

Daley, B. J., Shaw, C. R., Balistrieri, T., Glasenapp, I., & Placentine, L. (1999). Concept maps: A strategy to teach and evaluate critical thinking. *Journal of Nursing Education, 38*, 42–47.

Ennis, R. H. & Weir, E. (1985). *The Ennis-Weir critical thinking essay test.* Pacific Grove, CA: Midwest Publications.

Lunney, M. (2001). *Critical thinking & nursing diagnosis: Case studies & analysis.* Philadelphia: North American Nursing Diagnosis Association.

Lunney, M. (2003). Critical thinking and accuracy of nurses' diagnoses. *International Journal of Nursing Terminologies and Classifications, 14*(3), 96–107.

Mueller, A., Johnston, M., & Bligh, D. (2002). Joining mind mapping and care planning to enhance student critical thinking and achieve holistic nursing care. *Nursing Diagnosis, 13*(1), 24–27.

National League for Nursing Accrediting Commission. (2000). *Accreditation manual for post secondary, baccalaureate, and higher degree programs in nursing.* New York: Author.

National League for Nursing. (2004). *Critical thinking in clinical nursing practice-PN.* (Test Catalog). Retrieved August 11, 2004, from http://www.nln.org/testprods/index.htm.

NANDA International. (2005). *Nursing diagnoses: Definitions & classification 2005–2006.* Philadelphia: Author.

Nunnally, J. C. (2002). *Psychometric theory.* New York: McGraw-Hill.

Rubenfeld, M. G. & Scheffer, B. K. (1999). *Critical thinking in nursing: An interactive approach,* 2nd ed. Philadelphia: Lippincott.

Scheffer, B. K. & Rubenfeld, M. G. (2000). A consensus statement on critical thinking in nursing. *Journal of Nursing Education, 39*, 352–359.

Scheffer, B. K. (2001). Nurse educators' perspectives on their critical thinking. *Dissertation Abstracts International, 62*, 2B, p. 786 (ProQuest C., No. 3003400).

Senge, P. M. (1998, Summer). The practice of innovation. *Leader to Leader, 9,* 16–22. Retrieved July 21, 2004, from http://www.pfdf.org/leaderbooks/L2L/summer98/senge.html.

Staib, S. (2003). Teaching and measuring critical thinking. *Journal of Nursing Education, 42,* 498–508.

Stone, C. A., Davidson, L. J., Evans, J. L., & Hansen, M. A. (2001). Validity evidence for using a general critical thinking test to measure nursing students' critical thinking. *Holistic Nursing Practice, 15*(4), 65–74.

Tanner, C. A. (2005). What have we learned about critical thinking in nursing? *Journal of Nursing Education, 44*(2), 47–48.

Twibell, R., Ryan, M., & Hermiz, M. (2005). Faculty perceptions of critical thinking in student clinical experiences. *Journal of Nursing Education, 44*(2), 71–79.

Wheeler, L. A. & Collins, S. K. R. (2003). The influence of concept mapping on critical thinking in baccalaureate nursing students. *Journal of Professional Nursing, 19*(6), 339–345.

Critical Thinking Inventory

Critical Thinking Habits of the Mind

Confidence:

1. How do you justify your thinking to someone who questions your conclusions?

2. Under what circumstances do you second-guess your thinking?

3. Do you ever think aloud or do you wait to speak until you have your ideas firmly in place? Why?

4. In what situations are you easily swayed from your thinking by someone else's opinion?

Contextual Perspective:

1. Describe a situation where you are uncomfortable with ambiguity.

2. How often and under what circumstances do you ask questions that start with, "But, what if?"

3. How often and under what circumstances do you answer questions with "… it depends"?

4. When someone makes you angry, what do you consider as factors underlying that anger?

5. At what kind of tests are you best—those with multiple-choice questions or those with open-ended questions? Why?

6. When you tell a story, do you tend to include background information or keep more strictly to the point? Why?

Creativity:

1. In what creative activities do you engage that are not traditionally considered to be artistic, musical, etc.?

2. Do you feel more alike or different from most others? Explain how and why you feel that way.

3. If something doesn't work out as planned, are you most likely to give up (ranked as 1) or to see it as an opportunity to try a new approach (ranked as 10)? Where would you place yourself on this continuum of 1 to 10?

4. If you had to, which would you choose—living with lots of change or living with no change? Why?

5. Do you tend to see things the way other people do or are your interpretations often different from others? Give an example.

Flexibility:

1. How much of your daily life depends on habits? How much of your nursing practice depends on habits? Describe one habit in each of those areas of your life.

2. What is your initial reaction when things do not go as you planned?

3. Under what circumstances do you change your mind about your beliefs, feelings, assumptions?

4. How do you feel when the status quo is disrupted? How do you behave when this happens?

Inquisitiveness:

1. How do you respond to information you hear from authorities or read in a book?

2. Do you like to examine the reasons behind answers or do you like to be told the "correct" answer?

3. What is your first response when a speaker asks if anyone in the audience has questions?

4. Do people ever tell you to stop asking questions?

5. If your mind had compartments, would you see yours as having lots of walls, doors, or windows? Why? How many of each do you have?

6. How often during a day do you wonder "why"?

Intellectual Integrity:

1. How do you deal with ideas and information that conflict with your thinking?

2. How do you feel about debate on issues as opposed to having everyone agree? Why?

3. When you feel strongly about something, do you try to see the situation from the opposite view? How do you do that?

4. Describe your *feelings* and *thinking* when you receive constructive criticism.

Intuition:

1. How often do you have "gut" feelings, a "sixth sense," or a "premonition"?
2. How do you act upon those "feelings"?
3. How often do you say, "I should have gone with my first thought"?
4. On a scale of 1–10, with 10 being the highest, how would you rank your *intuition* skills as they relate to your personal life? To your nursing practice?

Open-mindedness:

1. How do you recognize where you have made assumptions as opposed to basing your conclusions on facts?
2. What are your assumptions (about cultures, health, illness, time, eating, exercise, economic status, education, and so forth) and how do they affect the questions you ask? The questions you don't ask? The conclusions you draw?
3. What are your "pet peeves" and how do you react when you encounter them?
4. How do you decide when you have enough information to draw a conclusion?
5. Do you characterize yourself as a liberal or conservative? If so, why do you characterize yourself that way?
6. Do you think other people see you as judgmental or not? Why?

Perseverance:

1. In what circumstances do you throw up your hands and say, "I give up!"
2. If you can't finish a task in the assigned time, do you rearrange things so you can devote more time to it, or do you say, "that's all the time I'll give to this."
3. Think of a time when you believed you demonstrated perseverance. What were the circumstances? Did you have to rack your brain to think of one or did you think of several immediately?
4. How often do other people say things like this to you: "I can't believe you kept at that!"

Reflection:

1. What phrases would you use to describe your thinking skills to new nursing students or staff?

2. How often do you go back and rethink something? Are there certain kinds of situations that you rethink more than others?

3. What things help and prevent you from reflecting on your thinking?

4. Describe yourself as seen through someone else's eyes.

5. What word or phrase would you put in this blank? I'm a _____ kind of thinker. Why did you choose that?

6. What parts of your thinking are strongest? Weakest?

7. What happens to your thinking when you are anxious, and what makes you anxious?

8. Describe how the following emotional states affect your thinking: love, hate, loneliness, frustration, sorrow, ecstasy, and so forth.

Critical Thinking Skills

Analyzing:

1. How do you organize your thinking about complex issues?

2. What goes on in your mind when situations seem overwhelming?

3. While solving problems, which are you more likely to do—get out paper and pencil to break it down, or talk it through in your head or out loud?

Applying Standards:

1. How do you decide if something is "right" or "wrong"?

2. When you are at work and someone is not doing her/his job as you think it should be done, what do you think and do?

3. How do you decide which authority is the highest?

Discriminating:

1. How do you decide what information is missing when you are problem-solving?

2. How often during a day do you ask questions such as these: "Could you be more specific?" "Can you give me more detail?"

3. When you walk into a room, what kinds of things do you see immediately?

4. Would you say you are a detail person or an idea person? Why?

5. What aids/instruments do you carry routinely to help you gather accurate data?

6. What techniques do you use to remember important information?

7. How did you learn to distinguish the nuances of assessment that allow you to customize/individualize patient care?

Information Seeking:

1. What are your five primary sources for finding accurate information? Have those changed over the past year? If so, how?

2. Is it easier to think about information after you hear it or after you see it, or both? What are the implications of this?

3. What kinds of information do you accept at "face value," and when do you believe it is necessary to validate and verify information?

4. How do you help people find answers when they ask you questions?

Logical Reasoning:

1. Do you prefer to solve problems in a sequential fashion, in a random, inspirational way, or in some combination of approaches?

2. When someone asks, "Why did you conclude that?" what is generally your response?

3. How do you decide when you have enough information to draw a conclusion?

4. Under what circumstances do you draw conclusions very quickly?

5. Under what circumstances do you tend to double-check things?

Predicting:

1. Describe how you project potentially positive and negative consequences of your decisions/actions, and also the decisions/actions of others.

2. How often during a day do you think, "What will happen if...?" In what circumstances do you ask that?

3. When caring for patients, how far into the future, on average, do you think?

Transforming Knowledge:

1. When you learn how to do something new, do you tend to memorize the steps or focus on the overall intent of the process?

2. Would you describe yourself as an abstract or concrete thinker? Explain.

3. When you learn something new, do you think about how you will use that information in different situations?

4. Describe an event in which you have drawn on knowledge from several different sources to deal with a problem.

Index of TACTICS

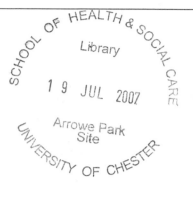

Index

Note: f = figure; t = table; b = box